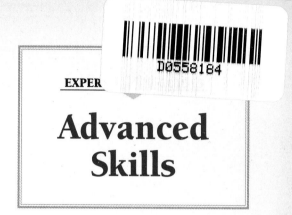

EXPER

Advanced Skills

Advanced Skills

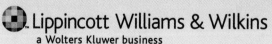 Lippincott Williams & Wilkins
a Wolters Kluwer business
Philadelphia · Baltimore · New York · London
Buenos Aires · Hong Kong · Sydney · Tokyo

STAFF

EXECUTIVE PUBLISHER
Judith A. Schilling McCann, RN, MSN

EDITORIAL DIRECTOR
William J. Kelly

CLINICAL DIRECTOR
Joan M. Robinson, RN, MSN

SENIOR ART DIRECTOR
Arlene Putterman

CLINICAL MANAGER
Collette Bishop Hendler, RN, BS, CCRN

EDITORIAL PROJECT MANAGER
Ann Houska

CLINICAL PROJECT MANAGER
Mary Perrong, RN, CRNP, MSN, APRN, BC

EDITORS
Lynne Christensen, Rita Doyle, Patricia Nale

CLINICAL EDITOR
Karen A. Hamel, RN, BSN

COPY EDITOR
Heather Ditch

DESIGNERS
ON-TRAK graphics, inc. (project manager), Linda J. Franklin

DIGITAL COMPOSITION SERVICES
Diane Paluba (manager), Joyce Rossi Biletz, Donna S. Morris

MANUFACTURING
Patricia K. Dorshaw (director), Beth J. Welsh

EDITORIAL ASSISTANTS
Megan L. Aldinger, Karen J. Kirk, Linda K. Ruhf

DESIGN ASSISTANT
Georg Purvis, 4th

INDEXER
Barbara Hodgson

© 2007 by Lippincott Williams & Wilkins. All rights reserved. This book is protected by copyright. No part of it may be reproduced, stored in a retrieval system, or transmitted, in any form or by any means—electronic, mechanical, photocopy, recording, or otherwise — without prior written permission of the publisher, except for brief quotations embodied in critical articles and reviews and testing and evaluation materials provided by publisher to instructors whose schools have adopted its accompanying textbook. Printed in the United States of America. For information, write Lippincott Williams & Wilkins, 323 Norristown Road, Suite 200, Ambler, PA 19002-2756.

LPNSkills010306

Library of Congress Cataloging-in-Publication Data

LPN expert guides. Advanced skills.
    p. ; cm.
  Includes bibliographical references and index.
   1. Practical nursing—Handbooks, manuals, etc. 2. Nursing—Handbooks, manuals, etc. I. Lippincott Williams & Wilkins. II. Title: Advanced skills.
   [DNLM: 1. Nursing Process—Handbooks. 2. Nursing Care—methods—Handbooks. 3. Nursing, Practical—methods—Handbooks. WY 49 L9232 2007]
RT62.L65 2007
610.73—dc22
ISBN 1-58255-831-0 (alk. paper)   2005034447

Contents

Contributors and consultants

Barbara C. Anderson, RN, BSN, MEd
Director
Virginia Beach (Va.) School of Practical Nursing

Dorothy Borton, RN, BSN, CIC
Infection Control Practitioner
Albert Einstein Healthcare Network
Philadelphia

Marie O. Brewer, RN
Clinical Compliance Auditor
Southeast Georgia Health System
Brunswick

Emilie M. Fedorov, RN, CS, MSN
Neuroscience Nurse Manager
Washoe Medical Center
Reno, Nev.

Linda J. Franklin, RN, BSN
Practical Nursing Instructor
Meridian Technology Center
Stillwater, Okla.

Donna M. Halloran-Krol, RN, BSN
Nursing Instructor
Ivy Tech State College
Valparaiso, Ind.

Karla Jones, RN, MS
Faculty–Department of Nursing
Treasure Valley Community College
Ontario, Ore.

Patricia B. Lisk, RN, BSN
Instructor
Augusta (Ga.) Technical College

Jennifer McWha, RN, MSN
Assistant Professor–Nursing Department
Del Mar College
Corpus Christi, Tex.

Lauren R. Roach, LPN, HCS-D
Manager of Office Operations
Good Samaritan Home Care Services
Vincennes, Ind.

Sherry Lee Rogman, RN
Staff-Charge Nurse Emergency Department
Bryan-LGH Medical Center
Lincoln, Nebr.

Bruce Austin Scott, APRN,BC, MSN
Nursing Instructor
San Joaquin Delta College
Stockton, Calif.

Georgia A. Simmons, RN, BSN
LPN Faculty
Ivy Tech State College
Madison, Ind.

1

ASSESSMENT

Obtaining a health history and performing a physical examination can be time-consuming, but completing them accurately and thoroughly is important. Try to collect patient data not only quickly but also systematically. To save time, cover several components at once. For example, make general observations while checking the patient's vital signs or asking history questions.

The health history and physical examination involve collecting two kinds of data: objective and subjective. Objective data are obtained through observation and are verifiable. For example, a red swollen arm in a patient with arm pain can be seen and verified by someone other than the patient. Subjective data are gathered from the patient's own account and can't be verified by anyone other than the patient; for example, when a patient says, "My head hurts" or "I have trouble sleeping at night."

This chapter presents the essential techniques for gathering information in the health history and physical examination.

Obtaining the health history

A health history gathers subjective data about the patient and explores previous and current problems. First, ask the patient about his general physical and emotional health, and then ask him about specific body systems and structures.

The accuracy and completeness of your patient's answers largely depend on your skill as an interviewer. Before you start asking questions, review the communication guidelines in the following sections.

HOW TO INTERVIEW THE PATIENT
Before asking your first question, you need to set the stage. Choose a quiet, private, well-lit, distraction-free interview setting; this will make it easier for you and your patient to interact and will help the

> ## Hints for communicating with the elderly
>
> An elderly patient may have sensory impairment, memory impairment, or a decreased attention span. If your patient is confused or has trouble communicating, you may need to rely on a family member for some or all of the health history.

patient feel more at ease. Make sure the patient is comfortable. Sit facing him, 3' to 4' (1 to 1.5 m) away.

Address the patient by a formal name, such as Mr. Jones or Ms. Carter. Don't call him by his first name unless he asks you to. Treating the patient with respect encourages him to trust you and give you accurate and complete information. Introduce yourself and explain that the purpose of the health history and physical examination is to identify his problem and provide information for planning care. Explain what you'll cover in the interview and how long it will last; then ask the patient to tell you what he expects from it. Speak slowly and clearly, using easy-to-understand language. Avoid medical terms and jargon. Reassure the patient that everything he says will be kept confidential. Watch the patient closely to see if he understands each question. If he doesn't seem to understand, repeat the question using different words or familiar examples.

Determine if the patient has a language barrier. For instance, does he speak and understand English? Most facilities have interpreters available to assist with English translations, or a member of the patient's family may be of help. Can the patient hear you? If your patient is hearing impaired, make sure the area is well lighted, face him, and speak slowly and clearly so that he can read your lips. If needed, see if your facility has a sign language interpreter available. When questioning an elderly patient, remember that he may have difficulty hearing or communicating. (See *Hints for communicating with the elderly*.)

Listen attentively and make eye contact frequently, but be aware that some patients—including Native Americans, Asians, and those from Arabic-speaking countries—may find eye contact disrespectful or aggressive. Use reassuring gestures, such as nodding your head, to encourage the patient to keep talking. (See *Pinpointing communication strategies*.)

Watch for nonverbal cues that indicate the patient is uncomfortable or unsure about how to answer a question. For example, he

Pinpointing communication strategies

The communication techniques in this table can help you make the most of your patient interview.

Silence	Moments of silence during the interview encourage the patient to continue talking and give you a chance to assess his ability to organize thoughts. You may find this technique difficult (most people are uncomfortable with silence), but the more you use it, the more comfortable you'll become.
Active listening	Active listening involves fully attending to the patient and being aware of the patient's emotional state. Active listening takes practice and also involves using verbal and nonverbal communication to encourage the patient to continue to speak.
Facilitation	Facilitation encourages the patient to continue with his story. Using such phrases as "please continue," "go on," or even "uh-huh" shows him that you're interested in what he's saying.
Confirmation	Confirmation ensures that you and the patient are on the same track. You might say, "If I understand you correctly, you said…" and then repeat the information the patient gave. This technique helps clear up misconceptions you or the patient might have.
Reflection	Reflection—or repeating something the patient has just said—can help you obtain more specific information. For example, a patient with a stomachache might say, "I know I have an ulcer." You might repeat, "You know you have an ulcer?" And the patient might then say, "Yes. I had one before and the pain is the same."
Clarification	Clarification is used to clear up confusing, vague, or misunderstood information. For example, if your patient says, "I can't stand this," your response might be, "What can't you stand?" or "What do you mean by 'I can't stand this'?" This gives the patient an opportunity to explain the statement.
Summary and conclusion	Summarizing, or restating, the information the patient gave you ensures that the data you've collected is accurate and complete. Summarizing also signals that the interview is about to end. Signaling the patient that you're ready to conclude the interview gives him the chance to gather his thoughts and make final pertinent statements. You can do this verbally by saying, "I think I have all the information I need now. Is there anything you'd like to add?"

Types of interview questions

Interview questions can be characterized as open-ended or closed.

OPEN-ENDED QUESTIONS
Open-ended questions require the patient to express feelings, opinions, and ideas. They also help you gather more information than can be gathered with closed questions. Open-ended questions encourage a good rapport with your patient because they show that you're interested in what he has to say. Examples of such questions include:
● Why did you come to the hospital tonight?
● How would you describe the problems you're having with your breathing?

● What lung problems, if any, do other members of your family have?

CLOSED QUESTIONS
Closed questions elicit yes-or-no answers or other one- or two-word responses. They limit the development of rapport with your patient. Closed questions can help you "zoom in" on specific points, but they don't give the patient the opportunity to elaborate. Examples of closed questions include:
● Do you ever get short of breath?
● Are you the only one in your family with lung problems?

---

might lower his voice or glance around uneasily. Be aware of your own nonverbal cues that might cause the patient to become uncomfortable. For example, if you cross your arms, you might appear "closed off" from him. If you stand while he's sitting, you might appear superior. If you glance at your watch, you might appear bored or rushed, which could keep him from answering questions completely.

Try using different types of questions. An open-ended question such as "How did you fall?" lets the patient respond more freely. The response can provide answers to many other questions. Closed questions are unlikely to provide extra information but might encourage the patient to give clear, concise feedback. (See *Types of interview questions*.)

Getting specific
Information gained from a health history forms the basis of the care plan. As with other nursing skills, your interviewing technique will improve with practice. To obtain a complete health history, gather information from each of the following categories, in sequence:
1. biographic data
2. chief complaint

Understanding an advance directive

The Patient Self-Determination Act lets a patient prepare an advance directive—a written document that states his wishes about health care if he becomes incapacitated or incompetent to make decisions. Elderly patients in particular may be interested in an advance directive because they tend to be concerned with end-of-life issues.

PROVIDING DIRECTION

If a patient doesn't have an advance directive in place, your health care facility must provide him with information about it and how to establish one.

An advance directive may include these details:

● the name of the person authorized by the patient to make medical decisions if the patient can no longer do so

● specific medical treatment the patient does or doesn't want
● instructions about pain medication and comfort; specifically, whether the patient wishes to receive certain treatment even if it may hasten his death
● information the patient wants to relay to his loved ones
● name of the patient's primary health care provider
● any other wishes.

3. medical history
4. family history
5. psychosocial history
6. activities of daily living.

BIOGRAPHIC DATA

Start the health history by obtaining biographic information from the patient: his name, address, telephone number, birth date, age, marital status, religion, and nationality. Find out who he lives with and the name and telephone number of a person to contact in case of an emergency. Other specific questions to ask include:

▪ Who's your primary physician? How do you get to the physician's office?
▪ Have you ever been treated before for your current problem?
▪ Do you have an advance directive? (See *Understanding an advance directive*.)

Your patient's answers to basic questions like these can offer important clues about personality, medical problems, and reliability. If he can't provide accurate information, ask him for the name of a friend or relative who can. Document who gave you the information.

CHIEF COMPLAINT

Try to pinpoint why the patient is seeking care at this time. To avoid misinterpretation, document this information in the patient's exact words. Here's what to ask:

■ What are your symptoms and when did they develop?

■ What prompted you to seek medical attention?

■ How have your symptoms affected your life and ability to function?

MEDICAL HISTORY

Ask the patient about past and current medical problems, such as hypertension, diabetes, or back pain. Typical questions include:

■ Have you ever been hospitalized? If so, when and for what reason?

■ Which childhood illnesses did you have?

■ Are you undergoing treatment for anything? If so, what's the treatment for and who's your physician?

■ Have you ever had surgery? If so, when and for what reason?

■ Are you allergic to anything in the environment, foods, latex or to any drugs? If so, what kind of allergic reaction do you have?

■ Are you taking medications, including over-the-counter preparations, such as aspirin, vitamins, and cough syrup? If so, how much do you take and how often? Do you use home remedies such as homemade ointments? Do you use herbal preparations or take dietary supplements? Do you use other alternative therapies, such as acupuncture, therapeutic massage, or chiropractic therapy?

FAMILY HISTORY

Ask the patient about his family's health to uncover whether he's at risk for certain illnesses. Typical questions include these:

■ Are your mother, father, and siblings living? If not, how old were they when they died? What was the cause of death?

■ Does your mother, father, or sibling have asthma, cancer, cataracts, diabetes, glaucoma, heart disease, hemophilia, high blood pressure, sickle cell anemia, or other illnesses?

PSYCHOSOCIAL HISTORY

Find out how the patient feels about himself, his place in society, and his relationships with others. Ask about occupation, education, financial status, and responsibilities. Here are some typical questions:

Asking about abuse

Abuse is a sensitive subject. Anyone can be a victim of abuse: a boyfriend or girlfriend, a spouse, an elderly patient, a child, or a parent. Also, abuse can come in many forms: physical, psychological, emotional, and sexual. When taking a patient's health history, ask two open-ended questions: When do you feel safe at home? When don't you feel safe?

OBSERVE THE REACTION

Even when you don't immediately suspect an abusive situation, be aware of how your patient reacts to these open-ended questions. Is the patient defensive, hostile, confused, or frightened? Determine how he interacts with you and others. Does he seem withdrawn or frightened or show other inappropriate behavior? Keep his reactions in mind while you perform the physical examination.

Remember, if the patient reports abuse of any kind to you, you're a mandated reporter. Inform the patient that you're obligated to report the abuse to the appropriate authorities.

- How have you coped with medical or emotional crises in the past? (See *Asking about abuse*.)
- Has your life changed recently? What changes in your personality or behavior have you noticed?
- Is the emotional support you receive from family and friends adequate?
- How often do you exercise? What types of things do you do to exercise? Do you walk, use a stationary bike, or lift weights? How often do you follow a healthful diet?
- How close do you live to health care facilities and are they easy to get to?
- Do you have health insurance?
- Are you on a fixed income with no extra money for health care?

ACTIVITIES OF DAILY LIVING

Find out what's normal for the patient by asking him to describe a typical day. Include diet and elimination; exercise and sleep; work and leisure; use of tobacco, alcohol, and other drugs; and religious observances.

- *Diet.* Ask the patient about his appetite, special diets, and food allergies. Can he afford to buy enough food? Who at his house cooks and shops?
- *Exercise and sleep.* Ask the patient if he has a special exercise program and, if so, why? Have him describe it. Ask how many hours

he sleeps at night, what his sleep pattern is like, and whether he feels rested after sleep.

■ *Work and leisure.* Ask the patient what he does for a living and what he does during leisure time. Does he have hobbies?

■ *Use of tobacco, alcohol, and other drugs.* Ask the patient if he smokes cigarettes. If so, how many does he smoke each day? Does he drink alcohol? If so, how much each day? Ask if he uses illicit drugs, such as marijuana or cocaine. If so, how often?

■ *Religious observances.* Ask the patient if he has religious beliefs that affect diet, dress, or health practices. Patients will feel reassured when you make it clear that you understand these points.

REVIEWING STRUCTURES AND SYSTEMS

The last part of the health history is a systematic review of the patient's body structures and systems. As you move into this phase of the history, find out about the patient's general condition by asking these questions:

■ What's your usual weight? Have you noticed that your clothes fit more loosely or tightly than usual?

■ Do you suffer from excess fatigue?

■ How many colds or other minor illnesses do you have each year?

■ Do you ever have unexplained episodes of fever, weakness, or night sweats?

■ Do you ever have trouble carrying out activities of daily living?

For the review of body structures and systems, always start at the top of the patient's head and work your way down his body, to ensure that you cover every area—the head-to-toe approach.

Here are some key questions to ask your patient about each body structure and system.

SKIN, HAIR, AND NAILS

Do you have a skin disease, such as psoriasis? Do you have rashes, scars, sores, or ulcers? Do you have any skin growths, such as warts, moles, tumors, or masses? Do you experience skin reactions to hot or cold weather?

Have you noticed any changes in the amount, texture, or character of your hair?

Have you noticed any changes in your nails? Do you have excessive nail splitting, cracking, or breaking?

HEAD

Do you get headaches? If so, where's the pain located and how intense is it? How often do the headaches occur, and how long do they last? Does anything trigger them, and how do you relieve them? Have you ever had a head injury? Do you have lumps or bumps on your head?

EYES, EARS, AND NOSE

When was your last eye examination? Do you wear glasses? Do you have glaucoma, cataracts, or color blindness? Does light bother your eyes? Do you have excessive tearing; blurred vision; double vision; or dry, itchy, burning, inflamed, or swollen eyes?

Do you have loss of balance, ringing in your ears, deafness, or poor hearing? Have you ever had ear surgery? If so, why and when? Do you wear a hearing aid? Do you have pain, swelling, or discharge from your ears? If so, has this problem occurred before and how frequently?

Have you ever had nasal surgery? If so, why and when? Have you ever had sinusitis or nosebleeds? Do you have nasal problems that cause breathing difficulties, frequent sneezing, or discharge?

MOUTH AND THROAT

Do you have mouth sores, a dry mouth, loss of taste, a toothache, or bleeding gums? Do you wear dentures, and if so, do they fit?

Do you have a sore throat, fever, or chills? How often do you get a sore throat, and have you seen a physician for this? Do you have difficulty swallowing? If so, is the problem with solids or liquids? Is it a constant problem or does it accompany sore throat or another problem? What, if anything, makes it go away?

NECK

Do you have swelling, soreness, lack of movement, stiffness, or pain in your neck? If so, did something specific cause it, such as too much exercise? How long have you had the problem? Does anything relieve it or aggravate it?

RESPIRATORY SYSTEM

Do you have shortness of breath on exertion or while lying in bed? How many pillows do you use at night? Do you have pain or wheezing when breathing? Do you have a productive cough? If so, what color is the sputum? Is it blood-tinged? Do you have night sweats?

Have you ever been treated for pneumonia, asthma, emphysema, or frequent respiratory tract infections? Have you ever had a chest X-ray or a tuberculin skin test? If so, when, and what were the results?

CARDIOVASCULAR SYSTEM

Do you have chest pain, palpitations, irregular heartbeat, fast heartbeat, shortness of breath, or a persistent cough? Have you ever had an electrocardiogram? If so, when?

Do you have high blood pressure, peripheral vascular disease, swelling of the ankles and hands, varicose veins, cold extremities, or intermittent pain in your legs?

BREASTS

Ask women these questions: Do you perform monthly breast self-examinations? When was your last clinical breast examination? Have you noticed a lump, a change in breast contour, breast pain, or discharge from your nipples? Have you ever had breast cancer? If not, has anyone else in your family had it? Have you ever had a mammogram? When, and what were the results?

Ask men these questions: Do you have pain in your breast tissue? Have you noticed lumps or a change in contour?

GI SYSTEM

Have you had nausea, vomiting, loss of appetite, heartburn, abdominal pain, frequent belching, or passing of gas? Have you lost or gained weight recently? How frequent are your bowel movements, and what color, odor, and consistency are your stools? Have you noticed a change in your regular pattern? Do you use laxatives frequently?

Have you had hemorrhoids, rectal bleeding, hernias, gallbladder disease, or a liver disease such as hepatitis?

URINARY SYSTEM

Do you have urinary problems, such as burning during urination, incontinence, urgency, retention, reduced urine flow, or dribbling? Do you get up during the night to urinate? If so, how many times? What color is your urine? Have you ever noticed blood in it? Have you been treated for kidney stones?

REPRODUCTIVE SYSTEM

Ask women these questions: How old were you when you started menstruating? How often do you get your period, and how long does it usually last? Do you have clots or pain? If you're post-menopausal, at what age did you stop menstruating? If you're in the transitional stage, what menopausal symptoms are you experiencing? Have you ever been pregnant? If so, how many times? What was the method of delivery? How many pregnancies resulted in live births? How many were miscarriages? Have you ever had an abortion?

What's your method of birth control? Are you involved in a long-term, monogamous relationship? Have you ever had a vaginal infection or a sexually transmitted disease? When was your last gynecologic examination and Papanicolaou test? What were the results?

Ask men these questions: Do you perform monthly testicular self-examinations? Have you ever had a prostate examination and, if so, when? Have you noticed penile pain, discharge, or lesions or testicular lumps? Which form of birth control do you use? Have you had a vasectomy? Are you involved in a long-term, monogamous relationship? Have you ever had a sexually transmitted disease?

MUSCULOSKELETAL SYSTEM

Do you have difficulty walking, sitting, or standing? Are you steady on your feet, or do you lose your balance easily? Do you have arthritis, gout, a back injury, muscle weakness, or paralysis?

NEUROLOGIC SYSTEM

Have you ever had seizures? Do you ever experience tremors, twitching, numbness, tingling, or loss of sensation in a part of the body? Are you less able to get around than you think you should be?

ENDOCRINE SYSTEM

Have you been unusually tired lately? Do you feel hungry or thirsty more than usual? Have you lost weight for unexplained reasons? How well can you tolerate heat or cold? Have you noticed changes in your hair texture or color? Have you been losing hair? Do you take hormonal medications?

HEMATOLOGIC SYSTEM

Have you ever been diagnosed with anemia or another blood abnormality? Do you bruise easily or become fatigued quickly? Have you ever had a blood transfusion?

EMOTIONAL STATUS

Do you ever experience mood swings or memory loss? Do you ever feel anxious, depressed, or unable to concentrate? Are you feeling unusually stressed? Do you ever feel unable to cope?

Performing the physical examination

After you've taken the patient's health history, proceed to the hands-on part, the physical examination. During the physical examination, you'll use all of your senses and a systematic approach to collect data about your patient's health. A complete physical examination includes a general survey, vital sign measurements, height and weight measurements, and examination of all organs and body systems. A head-to-toe approach is a systematic way of conducting the examination.

COLLECTING THE TOOLS

Before starting a physical examination, assemble the necessary tools, including cotton balls, gloves, a penlight, safety pins, and a stethoscope. (See *Examination tools*.)

Use a stethoscope with a diaphragm and a bell. The diaphragm has a flat, thin, plastic surface that picks up high-pitched sounds such as breath sounds. The bell has a smaller, open end that picks up low-pitched sounds, such as third and fourth heart sounds.

You'll need a penlight to illuminate the inside of the patient's nose and mouth, cast tangential light on lesions, and evaluate pupillary reactions.

Other tools include cotton balls and safety pins to test sensation and pain differentiation, and gloves to protect the patient and you.

Advanced practitioners use an ophthalmoscope to examine the internal structures of the eye, an otoscope to examine the external auditory canal and tympanic membrane, and a reflex hammer to evaluate deep tendon reflexes.

PERFORMING A GENERAL SURVEY

After assembling the necessary tools, move on to the first part of the physical examination: forming initial impressions of the patient, preparing him for the examination, and obtaining baseline data, including height, weight, and vital signs. This information will direct the rest of your examination.

Obtaining baseline data

Accurate measurements of your patient's height, weight, and vital signs provide critical information about the patient's body functions.

The first time you check a patient, record baseline vital signs and statistics. Afterward, take measurements at regular intervals, depending on the patient's condition and your facility's policy. A series of readings usually provides more valuable information than a single set. If you obtain an abnormal value, take the vital sign again to

Examination tools

Tools you'll use when performing the physical examination:

- blood pressure cuff
- cotton balls
- gloves
- examination gown and drape
- metric ruler (clear)
- near-vision and visual acuity charts
- penlight
- safety pins
- scale with height measurement
- stethoscope
- tape measure (cloth or paper)
- thermometer
- tuning fork
- wooden tongue blade.

make sure it's accurate. Remember that normal readings vary with the patient's age and from patient to patient.

HEIGHT AND WEIGHT

Height and weight are important for evaluating nutritional status, calculating medication dosages, and monitoring fluid loss or gain. Take the patient's baseline height and weight so you can gauge future weight changes or calculate medication dosages in an emergency.

BODY TEMPERATURE

Body temperature is measured in degrees Fahrenheit or degrees Celsius. Normal body temperature ranges from 96.7° to 100.5° F (35.9° to 38° C), depending on the route used for measurement.

Hyperthermia describes an oral temperature above 106° F (41.1° C); hypothermia describes a rectal temperature below 95° F (35° C).

To convert Celsius to Fahrenheit, multiply the Celsius temperature by 1.8 and add 32. To convert Fahrenheit to Celsius, subtract 32 from the Fahrenheit temperature and divide by 1.8.

PULSE

The patient's pulse reflects the amount of blood ejected with each heartbeat. To assess the pulse, palpate one of the patient's arterial pulse points and note the rate, rhythm, and amplitude (strength) of the pulse. A normal pulse for an adult is between 60 and 100 beats/minute. The radial pulse is the most easily accessible pulse site. However, in cardiovascular emergencies, the femoral or carotid pulse may be more appropriate because these sites are larger and closer to the heart and more accurately reflect the heart's activity.

Hypertension criteria

The seventh report of the Joint National Committee on Detection, Evaluation, and Treatment of High Blood Pressure recommends that hypertension be diagnosed when a higher-than-normal level has been found on two or more readings after the first screening. This table outlines the classification for adults age 18 and older.

CATEGORY	SYSTOLIC BLOOD PRESSURE (MM HG)		DIASTOLIC BLOOD PRESSURE (MM HG)
Normal	< 120	and	< 80
Prehypertension	120–139	or	80–89
Stage 1 hypertension	140–159	or	90–99
Stage 2 hypertension	≥ 160	or	≥ 100

If your patient has an irregular pulse, be sure to do the following:

■ Evaluate whether the irregularity follows a pattern.
■ Auscultate the apical pulse while palpating the radial pulse for 60 seconds. You should feel the pulse every time you hear a heartbeat.
■ Measure the pulse deficit—that is, the difference between the apical pulse rate and radial pulse rate. After you have this measurement, you can indirectly evaluate the ability of each cardiac contraction to eject sufficient blood into the peripheral circulation.
■ Evaluate pulse amplitude, or strength, using a numerical scale or descriptive term.

RESPIRATIONS

Along with counting respirations, note the depth and rhythm of each breath. A rate of 16 to 20 breaths/minute is normal for an adult. Observe the rhythm and symmetry of the chest wall as it expands during inspiration and relaxes during expiration. Be aware that skeletal deformity, fractured ribs, and collapsed lung tissue can cause unequal chest expansion. Note the use of accessory muscles or respiratory distress. Normal respirations are quiet and easy, so note abnormal sounds, such as wheezing or stridor.

BLOOD PRESSURE

Systolic and diastolic blood pressure readings are helpful in evaluating cardiac output, fluid and circulatory status, and arterial resistance. Normal systolic pressure is less than 120 mm Hg. Normal diastolic pressure is less than 80 mm Hg. (See *Hypertension criteria*.)

PHYSICAL EXAMINATION TECHNIQUES

During the physical examination, use drapes, exposing only the area to be examined. Develop a pattern for your examination, starting with the same body system and proceeding in the same sequence. Organize your steps to minimize the number of times the patient needs to change position. By using the head-to-toe approach, you'll also be less likely to forget an area.

Four techniques are used in the physical examination: inspection, palpation, percussion, and auscultation. The techniques are used in sequence, except when performing an abdominal assessment. Because palpation and percussion can alter bowel sounds, the sequence for assessing the abdomen is inspection, auscultation, percussion, and palpation. Let's look at each technique in the sequence, one at a time.

Inspection

Inspect the patient using seeing, smelling, and hearing to check for normal conditions and deviations. Performed correctly, inspection can reveal more than other techniques.

Inspection begins when you first meet the patient and continues throughout the health history and physical examination. As you exam each body system, check for color, size, location, movement, texture, symmetry, odors, and sounds.

Palpation

Palpation requires you to touch the patient with different parts of your hand, using varying degrees of pressure. To do this, you need short fingernails and warm hands. Always palpate tender areas last. Tell your patient what you're palpating and why.

Don't forget to wear gloves, especially when palpating mucous membranes or other areas where you might come in contact with body fluids.

As you palpate each body system, evaluate the following features:

■ texture—rough or smooth?
■ temperature—warm, hot, or cold?
■ moisture—dry, wet, or moist?

■ motion—still or vibrating?
■ consistency of structures—solid or fluid filled?

Percussion

Percussion involves tapping the fingers quickly and sharply against parts of the patient's body, usually the chest or abdomen. The technique is used to locate organ borders, identify organ shape and position, and determine if an organ is solid or filled with fluid or gas. Percussion requires a skilled touch and an ear trained to detect slight variations in sound. Organs and tissues produce sounds of varying loudness, pitch, and duration, depending on their density. For instance, air-filled cavities, such as the lungs, produce markedly different sounds from those produced by the liver and other dense tissues.

Auscultation

Auscultation, usually the last step, involves listening for various breath, heart, and bowel sounds with a stethoscope. To prevent the spread of infection among patients, clean the heads and end pieces with alcohol or a disinfectant. Your stethoscope should have snugly fitting ear plugs, which you'll position toward your nose; tubing no longer than 15″ (38.1 cm), with an internal diameter not greater than ⅛″ (0.3 cm); a diaphragm; and a bell.

HOW TO AUSCULTATE

Hold the diaphragm firmly against the patient's skin, enough to leave a slight ring afterward. Hold the bell lightly against his skin, enough to form a seal. (Holding the bell too firmly causes the skin to act as a diaphragm, obliterating low-pitched sounds.)

Hair on the patient's chest may cause friction on the end piece, which can mimic abnormal breath sounds such as crackles. You can minimize this problem by lightly dampening the hair before auscultating.

Also, keep these points in mind:
■ Provide a quiet environment.
■ Make sure the area to be auscultated is exposed. Don't try to auscultate over a gown or bed linens because they can interfere with sounds.
■ Warm the stethoscope head in your hand.
■ Close your eyes to help focus your attention.
■ Listen to and try to identify the characteristics of one sound at a time.

HEAD-TO-TOE EXAMINATION: NORMAL FINDINGS

To distinguish between health and disease, you must be able to recognize normal findings in each part of the body. When you perform a physical examination, use this head-to-toe roster of normal findings as a reference. It's designed to help you quickly zero in on physical abnormalities and evaluate your patient's overall condition.

GENERAL SURVEY

■ Alert and oriented; responds appropriately
■ Coherent speech
■ Intact memory (remote and recent)
■ Well-groomed and well-nourished
■ Smooth gait; no involuntary movements
■ Vital signs, height, and weight within normal range for age-group

SKIN
Inspection

■ Color varying from pink to dark brown, depending on ethnic background
■ No pallor, jaundice, cyanosis, bruising, erythema, rashes, or lesions
■ Normal hair texture and distribution
■ Nail bed color varying from pink to brown depending on skin color
■ Angle of nail base 160 degrees or less; no clubbing (see *Checking for clubbed fingers,* page 18)

Palpation

■ Smooth texture, and warm, dry skin
■ Normal turgor or elasticity (skin quickly returns to original shape when gently squeezed)

LIFE STAGES Decreased turgor occurs with dehydration and aging. In an elderly patient, the skin of the forearm tends to be paper-thin, dry, and wrinkled, so it doesn't accurately represent the patient's hydration status. To accurately determine skin turgor in an elderly patient, try squeezing the skin of the sternum or forehead instead of the forearm.

HEAD AND NECK
Inspection
HEAD

■ A symmetrical, lesion-free skull

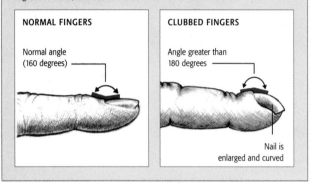

Checking for clubbed fingers

To assess the patient for chronic tissue hypoxia, check his fingers for clubbing. Normally, the angle between the fingernail and the point where the nail enters the skin is about 160 degrees. Clubbing occurs when that angle increases to 180 degrees or more, as shown below.

NORMAL FINGERS

Normal angle
(160 degrees)

CLUBBED FINGERS

Angle greater than
180 degrees

Nail is
enlarged and curved

■ Symmetrical facial structures with normal variations in skin texture and pigmentation
■ An ability to shrug the shoulders, a sign of an adequately functioning cranial nerve XI (accessory nerve)

NECK
■ Unrestricted range of motion in the neck
■ No bulging of the thyroid
■ Symmetrical lymph nodes with no swelling
■ Flat jugular veins

Palpation
HEAD
■ No lumps or tenderness on the head
■ Symmetrical strength in the facial muscles, a sign of adequately functioning cranial nerves V and VII (trigeminal and facial nerves)
■ Symmetrical sensation when you stroke a wisp of cotton on each cheek

NECK
■ Mobile, soft lymph nodes less than ½" (1.3 cm) with no tenderness

- Symmetrical pulses in the carotid arteries
- A palpable, symmetrical, lesion-free thyroid with no tenderness
- Midline location of the trachea and absence of tracheal tenderness
- No crepitus, tenderness, or lesions in the cervical spine
- Symmetrical muscle strength in the neck

EYES
Inspection
- No edema, scaling, or lesions on eyelids
- Eyelids completely covering corneas when closed
- Symmetrical, lesion-free upper eyelids that don't sag or droop when the patient opens his eyes
- Evenly distributed eyelashes that curve outward
- Globe of the eye neither protruding from nor sunken into the orbit
- Eyebrows with equal size, color, and distribution
- Absence of nystagmus
- Clear conjunctiva with visible small blood vessels and no signs of drainage
- White sclera visible through the conjunctiva
- A transparent anterior chamber that contains no visible material when you shine a penlight into the side of the eye
- Transparent, smooth, and bright cornea with no visible irregularities or lesions
- Closing of the lids of both eyes when you stroke each cornea with a wisp of cotton, a test of cranial nerve V (trigeminal nerve)
- Round, equal-sized pupils that react to light and accommodation
- Constriction of both pupils when you shine a light on one
- Lacrimal structures free from exudate, swelling, and excessive tearing
- Proper eye alignment
- Parallel eye movement in each of the six cardinal fields of gaze

Palpation
- No eyelid swelling or tenderness
- Lacrimal sacs that don't regurgitate fluid

EARS
Inspection
- Bilaterally symmetrical, proportionately sized auricles
- Color match between the ears and facial skin
- No signs of inflammation, lesions, or nodules

- No cracking, thickening, scaling, or lesions behind the ear when you bend the auricle forward
- No visible discharge from the auditory canal
- A patent external meatus
- Skin color on the mastoid process that matches the skin color of the surrounding area
- No redness or swelling

Palpation

- No masses or tenderness on the auricle
- No tenderness on the auricle or tragus during manipulation
- Either small, nonpalpable lymph nodes on the auricle or discrete, mobile lymph nodes with no signs of tenderness
- Well-defined, bony edges on the mastoid process with no signs of tenderness

NOSE AND MOUTH
Inspection
NOSE

- Symmetrical, lesion-free nose with no deviation of the septum or discharge
- Little or no nasal flaring
- Nonedematous frontal and maxillary sinuses
- Ability to identify familiar odors
- No visible lesions and no purulent drainage

MOUTH

- Pink lips with no dryness, cracking, lesions, or cyanosis
- Symmetrical facial structures
- Ability to purse the lips and puff out the cheeks, a sign of an adequately functioning cranial nerve VII (facial nerve)
- Ability to open and close the mouth easily
- Light pink, moist oral mucosa with no ulcers or lesions
- Visible salivary ducts with no inflammation
- White, hard palate
- Pink, soft palate
- Pink gums with no tartar, inflammation, hemorrhage, or leukoplakia
- All teeth intact, with no signs of occlusion, caries, or breakage
- Pink tongue that protrudes symmetrically and has no swelling, coating, ulcers, or lesions
- Ability to move the tongue easily and without tremor, a sign of a properly functioning cranial nerve XII (hypoglossal nerve)

- No lesions or inflammation on the posterior pharynx
- Lesion-free tonsils that are the appropriate size for the patient's age
- A uvula that moves upward when the patient says "ah" and a gag reflex that occurs when a tongue blade touches the posterior pharynx. These are signs of properly functioning cranial nerves IX and X.

Palpation
NOSE
- No structural deviation, tenderness, or swelling on the external nose
- No tenderness or edema on the frontal and maxillary sinuses

MOUTH
- Lips free from pain and induration
- No tenderness on the posterior and lateral surfaces of the tongue
- No tenderness or nodules on the floor of the mouth

THORAX AND LUNGS
Inspection
- Symmetrical side-to-side configuration of the chest
- Anteroposterior diameter less than the transverse diameter, with a 1:2 ratio in an adult
- Normal chest shape, with no deformities, such as a barrel chest, kyphosis, retraction, sternal protrusion, or depressed sternum
- Costal angle less than 90 degrees, with the ribs joining the spine at a 45-degree angle
- Quiet, unlabored respirations with no use of accessory neck, shoulder, or abdominal muscles. You should also see no intercostal, substernal, or supraclavicular retractions.
- Symmetrically expanding chest wall during respirations
- Normal adult respiratory rate of 12 to 20 breaths/minute, with some variation depending on the patient's age
- Regular respiratory rhythm, with expiration taking about twice as long as inspiration. Men and children breathe diaphragmatically, whereas women breathe thoracically.
- Skin color that matches the rest of the body's complexion

Palpation
- Warm, dry skin
- No tender spots or bulges in the chest

Auscultation sequence

Follow the auscultation sequence below when you listen to the patient's lungs. Remember to compare sounds on one side with those on the other as you proceed.

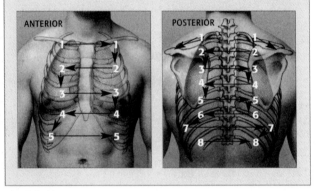

Auscultation
- Loud, high-pitched bronchial breath sounds over the trachea (see *Auscultation sequence*)
- Intense, medium-pitched bronchovesicular breath sounds over the mainstem bronchi, between the scapulae, and below the clavicles
- Soft, breezy, low-pitched vesicular breath sounds over most of the peripheral lung fields (see *Qualities of normal breath sounds*)
- No adventitious sounds (see *Abnormal breath sounds*)

HEART
Inspection
- No visible pulsations, except at the point of maximum impulse (PMI)

Palpation
- No detectable vibrations or thrills
- No pulsations, except at the PMI and epigastric area (At the PMI, a localized (less than ½" [1.3 cm] in diameter) tapping pulse may be felt at the start of systole. In the epigastric area, pulsation from the abdominal aorta may be palpable.)

Qualities of normal breath sounds

Use this table as a quick reference for the qualities of normal breath sounds.

BREATH SOUND	QUALITY	LOCATION
Tracheal	Harsh, high-pitched	Over trachea
Bronchial	Loud, high-pitched	Next to trachea
Bronchovesicular	Medium loudness and pitch	Next to sternum
Vesicular	Soft, low-pitched	Remainder of lungs

Abnormal breath sounds

Here's a quick guide to the different types of abnormal breath sounds.

SOUND	DESCRIPTION
Crackles	Light crackling, popping, intermittent nonmusical sounds—like hairs being rubbed together—heard on inspiration or expiration
Pleural friction rub	Low-pitched, continual, superficial, squeaking or grating sound—like pieces of sandpaper being rubbed together—heard on inspiration and expiration
Rhonchi	Low-pitched, monophonic snoring sounds heard primarily on expiration but also throughout the respiratory cycle
Stridor	High-pitched, monophonic crowing sound heard on inspiration; louder in the neck than in the chest wall
Wheezes	High-pitched, continual musical or whistling sound heard primarily on expiration but sometimes also on inspiration

Auscultation

■ First heart sound (S$_1$)—the *lub* sound; heard best with the diaphragm of the stethoscope over the mitral area with the patient in a left lateral position. It sounds longer, lower, and louder there than the second heart sound (S_2). S_1 splitting may be heard in the tricuspid area. S_1 sound is split when closure of the tricuspid valve is delayed.

■ Second heart sound (S_2)—the *dub* sound; heard best with the diaphragm of the stethoscope over the aortic area with the patient sitting and leaning forward. It sounds shorter, sharper, higher, and louder there than the S_1 sound. Normal S_2 splitting may be heard in the pulmonic area on inspiration. S_2 sound is split when closure of pulmonic valve is delayed.

■ Third heart sound (S_3)—heard best with the bell of the stethoscope over the mitral area with the patient in a supine position and exhaling. It sounds short, dull, soft, and low.

LIFE STAGES This sound is normal in children and slender, young adults with no cardiovascular disease. It usually disappears between ages 25 and 35. However, in an older adult it may signify ventricular failure.

■ Murmurs—Innocent murmurs are soft and short, and they vary with respirations and patient position. They occur in early systole and are heard best in the pulmonic or mitral area with the patient in a supine position.

LIFE STAGES A heart murmur may be functional in children and young adults but is abnormal in older adults.

ABDOMEN
Inspection

■ Skin free from vascular lesions, jaundice, surgical scars, and rashes
■ Faint venous patterns (except in thin patients)
■ Flat, round, or scaphoid abdominal contour
■ Symmetrical abdomen
■ Umbilicus positioned midway between the xiphoid process and the symphysis pubis, with a flat or concave hemisphere
■ No variations in skin color
■ No apparent bulges
■ Abdominal movement apparent with respirations
■ Pink or silver-white striae from pregnancy or weight loss

Auscultation

■ High-pitched, gurgling bowel sounds, heard every 5 to 15 seconds through the diaphragm of the stethoscope in all four quadrants of the abdomen
■ Vascular sounds heard through the bell of the stethoscope
■ Venous hum over the inferior vena cava

■ No bruits, murmurs, friction rubs, or other venous hums

Palpation, light
■ No tenderness or masses
■ Abdominal musculature free from tenderness and rigidity
■ No guarding, distention, or ascites

EXTREMITIES
Inspection
■ No gross deformities
■ Symmetrical body parts
■ Good body alignment
■ Full range of motion in all muscles and joints
■ No pain with full range of motion
■ No visible swelling or inflammation of joints or muscles
■ Equal bilateral limb length and symmetrical muscle mass

Palpation
■ Normal shape with no swelling or tenderness
■ Equal bilateral muscle tone, texture, and strength
■ No involuntary contractions or twitching
■ Equally strong bilateral pulses

DOCUMENTATION
■ When you're finished with your examination, document your findings on the appropriate form.
■ Document general information.
■ Record findings by body system to organize the information and use anatomic landmarks in your descriptions.

2

INFECTION CONTROL

The Centers for Disease Control and Prevention (CDC) and the Healthcare Infection Control Practices Advisory Committee (HICPAC) have developed guidelines for isolation precautions in hospitals. These guidelines have two levels of precautions:

- Standard precautions
- Transmission-based precautions, which are further divided into airborne precautions, contact precautions, and droplet precautions

STANDARD PRECAUTIONS

Standard precautions are designed to decrease the risk of transmission of microorganisms from recognized and unrecognized sources of infection. These precautions should be followed at all times with every patient. According to the CDC and HICPAC, blood, body fluids, secretions and excretions (except sweat), nonintact skin, and mucous membranes should be handled as if they contain infectious agents, regardless of the patient's diagnosis. Standard precautions are to be used in conjunction with other transmission-based precautions.

CONTRAINDICATIONS
None known.

EQUIPMENT
Gloves • masks • goggles or face shields • gowns or aprons • resuscitation bag • bags for specimens • Environmental Protection Agency (EPA)-registered tuberculocidal disinfectant, diluted bleach solution (diluted between 1:10 and 1:100, mixed fresh daily), or both • EPA-registered disinfectant labeled effective against hepatitis B virus (HBV) and human immunodeficiency virus (HIV)

ESSENTIAL STEPS

- Wash your skin immediately if it becomes contaminated with blood or body fluids, excretions, secretions, or drainage.
- Wash your hands before and after patient care and after removing gloves.
- You may use an alcohol-based hand rub for routine decontamination if your hands aren't visibly soiled.
- Wear gloves if you may come in contact with blood, specimens, tissue, body fluids, secretions or excretions, mucous membrane, broken skin, or contaminated surfaces or objects. (See *Choosing the right gloves,* page 28.)
- Change your gloves and wash your hands between patient contacts.
- Wear a fluid-resistant gown, face shield or goggles, and a mask during procedures likely to cause splashing of blood or body fluids (such as surgery, endoscopic procedures, or assisting with intubation or suctioning).
- You may wear additional personal protective equipment, such as shoe covers, if you may be exposed to large amounts of blood or body fluids (such as in trauma care).
- Handle used needles and other sharp instruments carefully. Don't bend, break, or reinsert them into their original sheaths (use the single-handed recapping technique when recapping is necessary); don't remove needles from syringes; and don't handle these items unnecessarily. Activate any safety mechanism immediately after use. Discard needles and other sharp instruments intact immediately after use into a puncture-resistant disposal box.
- Use tools to pick up broken glass or other sharp objects.
- Use a needleless I.V. system, if available.
- Immediately notify your employer of all needle-stick or other sharp-object injuries, mucosal splashes, or contamination of open wounds or nonintact skin with blood or body fluids.
- Label all specimens collected from patients and place them in plastic bags at the collection site. Attach completed requisition slips to the outside of bags and send the specimens to the lab immediately.
- Place all items that have come in direct contact with the patient's secretions, excretions, blood, drainage, or body fluids in a single impervious bag or container before removing them from the room.
- Place linens and trash in single bags of sufficient thickness to contain the contents.

Choosing the right gloves

Allergic reactions may result from cumulative exposure to latex gloves and other products that contain latex. Patients may also have latex sensitivity.

Take these steps to protect you and your patient from allergic reactions to natural rubber latex:

● Use nonlatex (vinyl or synthetic) gloves for activities not likely to involve contact with infectious materials (such as food preparation and routine cleaning).

● You may wear nonlatex gloves for brief activities, even if contact with infectious material is possible.

● Use appropriate barrier protection when handling infectious materials. If you choose latex gloves, use powder-free gloves with reduced protein content. Powder in any gloves is very drying to skin and may cause greater risk of exposure to skin if skin is dry and cracked.

● After wearing and removing gloves, wash your hands with soap and dry them thoroughly.

● When wearing latex gloves, don't use oil-based hand creams or lotions unless they'll maintain glove barrier protection.

● Refer to the material safety data sheet for the appropriate gloves to wear when handling chemicals.

● Learn latex allergy prevention and know the symptoms of latex allergy: skin rash, hives, flushing, itching, asthma, shock, and nasal, eye, or sinus symptoms.

● If your patient has a latex allergy, make sure that his environment is latex free and that health care providers who come in contact with the patient are alerted to his allergy.

● If you suspect you have a latex allergy, use nonlatex gloves, avoid contact with products that contain latex, and consult a physician experienced in treating latex allergy. Report problems to your supervisor, and follow your facility's policy for evaluation.

If you're allergic to latex:

● Avoid contact with latex gloves and other products that contain latex.

● Avoid areas where you might inhale powder from latex gloves worn by other workers.

● Inform your employer and your health care providers.

● Wear a medical identification bracelet.

● Follow your physician's instructions for dealing with latex reactions.

● Check packages, trays, and kits for items containing latex. (Products containing natural rubber latex must be labeled clearly on the exterior.)

■ While wearing appropriate personal protective equipment, promptly clean all blood and body fluid spills. Blot the spill with paper towels or other absorbent material; then, clean the spill area with detergent and water. Finally, if the area hasn't been contaminated by agents or concentrations of agents for which higher-level disinfection is recommended, clean it with an EPA-registered tuberculocidal disinfectant, a bleach solution diluted between 1:10 and 1:100 (mixed daily), or an EPA-registered disinfectant labeled effective against HBV and HIV. Contact building or environmental services, according to your facility's policy, for larger spills.

■ If you have an exudative lesion, avoid all patient contact until the condition has resolved and you've been cleared by your employer's health care provider.

■ If you have broken skin on your hands, even though you should wear gloves, avoid situations that may bring you in contact with blood and body fluids until the condition has resolved and you've been cleared by your employer's health care provider.

SPECIAL CONSIDERATIONS

■ Hand hygiene and appropriate use of personal protective equipment should be routine infection control practices (see *Defining hand hygiene,* page 30)

■ Keep mouthpieces, resuscitation bags, and other ventilation devices nearby to eliminate the need for emergency mouth-to-mouth resuscitation.

 RED FLAG You may not know what organisms are present in every situation; use standard precautions for every contact with blood, body fluids, secretions, excretions, drainage, mucous membranes, and nonintact skin.

■ Use your judgment in individual cases about when to obtain an order to use enhanced isolation precautions, such as airborne, contact, or droplet precautions.

■ If your work requires you to be exposed to blood, you should receive the HBV vaccine series. You should have titers drawn periodically and be monitored to determine if you need an HBV booster.

COMPLICATIONS

Failure to follow standard precautions may lead to exposure to blood-borne diseases or other infections and to the complications they may cause.

DOCUMENTATION

■ Record special needs for transmission-based precautions.

■ Record standard precaution measures taken per facility policy.

Defining hand hygiene

In 2002, the Centers for Disease Control and Prevention (CDC) published its Guideline for Hand Hygiene in Health Care Settings. Hand hygiene covers hand washing, antiseptic hand washing, surgical hand antisepsis, and antiseptic hand rubs or sanitizers.

HAND WASHING

Redefined by the CDC guideline, hand washing refers to washing the hands with plain (such as nonantimicrobial) soap and water. For antiseptic hand washing, an antiseptic agent (such as chlorhexidine, triclosan, or iodophor) is used. Surgical personnel perform surgical hand antisepsis preoperatively to eliminate transient bacteria and reduce resident hand flora.

Hand washing is appropriate whenever the hands are soiled or contaminated with infectious material. Whether it involves plain soap and water or an antiseptic, hand washing is still the single most effective method for preventing the spread of infection.

HAND RUBS

Hand hygiene also includes the use of antiseptic hand rubs or sanitizers, also called waterless antiseptic agents because no water is required. These products are appropriate for decontaminating the hands after minimal contamination. An antiseptic alcohol-containing product designed to reduce the number of viable microorganisms on the skin is applied and rubbed in until the product has dried (usually within 30 seconds). These hand rubs usually contain emollients to prevent skin drying and chapping.

TRANSMISSION-BASED PRECAUTIONS

Whenever a patient is known or suspected to be infected with highly contagious or epidemiologically important pathogens transmitted by air, droplet, or contact with skin or other contaminated surfaces, follow transmission-based precautions along with standard precautions. One or more types of transmission-based precautions may be combined and followed when a patient has a disease—or more than one disease—with multiple routes of transmission.

Airborne precautions

Used along with standard precautions, airborne precautions prevent the spread of infectious diseases transmitted by pathogens that are breathed, sneezed, or coughed. (See *Diseases requiring airborne precautions,* page 32.) Effective airborne precautions require a negative air–pressure room with the door closed to maintain air pressure balance between the isolation room and adjoining anteroom, hallway, or corridor. Negative air pressure must be monitored and air vented to the outside of the building or filtered through high-efficiency particulate air (HEPA) filtration before recirculation. Everyone entering the patient's room must wear a disposable or reusable respirator.

RED FLAG The disposable or reusable respirator must be fit to the face properly each time it's worn.

CONTRAINDICATIONS
None known.

EQUIPMENT
Disposable N95 or HEPA respirators or reusable HEPA respirators or powered air-purifying respirator (PAPR) ● surgical masks ● isolation door card ● thermometer ● stethoscope ● blood pressure cuff ● personal protective equipment, as needed

PREPARATION OF EQUIPMENT
■ Keep airborne precaution supplies on cart outside isolation room.

ESSENTIAL STEPS
■ Situate the patient in a negative-pressure room with door closed. There should be an anteroom if possible.
■ Put an "airborne precautions" sign on the door to notify anyone entering the room and on the patient's chart to notify other departments that may come in contact with the patient. Check your facility's policy to determine proper signage.
■ Keep the patient's door (and the anteroom door, if appropriate) closed, to maintain negative pressure and contain airborne pathogens.
■ Monitor negative air pressure.
■ Pick up and put on the respirator, according to manufacturer's directions.
■ Adjust the straps for a firm, comfortable fit.

Diseases requiring airborne precautions

DISEASE	PRECAUTIONARY PERIOD
Avian influenza A (H5N1)	For 14 days after start of symptoms, or until alternative diagnosis is confirmed
Chickenpox (varicella)	Until lesions are crusted and no new lesions appear
Disseminated herpes zoster	For duration of illness
Localized herpes zoster in immunocompromised patients	For duration of illness
Measles (rubeola)	For duration of illness
Monkeypox	Until all lesions are crusted
Pulmonary or laryngeal tuberculosis (TB), confirmed or suspected	After patient has started effective therapy, his condition is improving (decreased cough and fever and improved chest X-ray findings), and three consecutive sputum smears collected on different days are negative for TB; or TB is ruled out
Severe acute respiratory syndrome (SARS)	For duration of illness
Smallpox (variola major)	For duration of illness and until all scabs fall off
Viral hemorrhagic infections (Ebola, Lassa, Marburg)	For duration of illness with severe pulmonary involvement, or when patient is undergoing aerosolized treatment or procedures that induce cough

■ Check the fit and respiratory seal. (See *Respirator seal check.*)
■ Tape an impervious bag to the patient's bedside for disposal of facial tissues.
■ Make sure visitors wear respirators while in the room.
■ Limit the patient's movement from the room.
■ Make sure the patient wears a surgical mask over his nose and mouth when he leaves the room.

Respirator seal check

Before using a respirator, always check the respirator seal. To do this, place both of your hands over the respirator and exhale. If air leaks around your nose, adjust the nosepiece. If air leaks at the respirator's edges, adjust the straps along the side of your head. Recheck respirator fit after this adjustment.

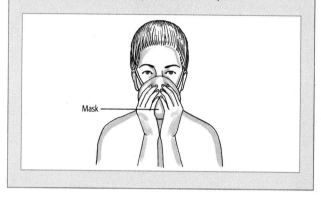

Mask

■ Notify the receiving department of airborne isolation precautions so they can be maintained and the patient can be returned to the room promptly.

SPECIAL CONSIDERATIONS

■ Before leaving the room, remove gloves (if worn) and wash your hands.

🏴 *RED FLAG Strict hand washing is required after contact with the patient or items contaminated with respiratory secretions.*

■ Remove respirator outside the room after closing door.

■ Discard respirator or clean and store it until next use; follow facility policy and manufacturer's recommendations.

■ To prevent microbial growth, store nondisposable respirators in dry, well-ventilated place (not plastic bag).

■ Two patients with the same infection may share a room, if necessary.

■ Reinforce the explanation of the isolation precautions to the patient and his family.

■ Staff or visitors with no history of specific disease or no vaccination against it shouldn't enter the room or provide care.

■ Reinforce infection control techniques, such as good hand washing, with the patient and his family.

COMPLICATIONS
None known.

DOCUMENTATION
■ Record the need for airborne precautions, as indicated by facility.
■ Document the dates airborne precautions were started and maintained.
■ Describe the patient's tolerance of precautions.
■ Document reinforced teaching of the patient and family.
■ Record the date precautions were stopped.
■ Document microbiology and virology specimens obtained and results of laboratory tests if available.

Contact precautions

Contact precautions prevent the spread of infectious diseases transmitted by direct or indirect contact with body substances or contaminated items or surfaces containing infectious agents. Contact precautions are used with patients infected or colonized (microorganisms present but signs or symptoms of infection absent) with epidemiologically important organisms. (See *Diseases requiring contact precautions.*) Effective contact precautions require a private room or cubicle and the use of gloves and gowns by anyone having contact with the patient, the patient's support equipment, or items soiled with body substances containing the infectious agent. Thorough hand washing and proper handling and disposal of articles contaminated by the body substance containing the infectious agent are also essential.

CONTRAINDICATIONS
None known.

EQUIPMENT
Gloves ● gowns or aprons ● masks, if necessary ● isolation door card ● plastic bags ● thermometer ● stethoscope ● blood pressure cuff

PREPARATION OF EQUIPMENT
■ Keep all contact precaution supplies outside the patient's room in a cart or anteroom.

Diseases requiring contact precautions

DISEASE	PRECAUTIONARY PERIOD
Acute viral (acute hemorrhagic) conjunctivitis	For duration of illness
Avian influenza A (H5N1)	For 14 days after start of symptoms, or until an alternative diagnosis is confirmed
Clostridium difficile enteric infection	For duration of illness
Cutaneous diphtheria	For duration of illness
Enteroviral infection, in diapered or incontinent patients	For duration of illness
Escherichia coli disease, in diapered or incontinent patients	For duration of illness
Hepatitis A, in diapered or incontinent patients	For duration of illness
Herpes simplex virus infection (neonatal or mucocutaneous)	For duration of illness
Impetigo	Until 24 hours after start of effective therapy
Infection or colonization with multidrug-resistant bacteria	Until antibiotic therapy ends and culture is negative
Major abscesses, cellulitis, or pressure ulcer	Until 24 hours after start of effective therapy
Monkeypox	Until all lesions are crusted
Parainfluenza virus infection, in diapered or incontinent patients	For duration of illness
Pediculosis (lice)	Until 24 hours after start of effective therapy
Respiratory syncytial virus infection, in infants and young children	For duration of illness

(continued)

Diseases requiring contact precautions (*continued*)

DISEASE	PRECAUTIONARY PERIOD
Rotavirus infection, in diapered or incontinent patients	For duration of illness
Rubella, congenital syndrome	During any hospitalization until infant is 1 year old, unless nasopharyngeal and urine cultures are negative after age 3 months
Scabies	Until 24 hours after start of effective therapy
Severe acute respiratory syndrome	For duration of illness
Shigellosis, in diapered or incontinent patients	For duration of illness
Smallpox	For duration of illness
Staphylococcal furunculosis, in infants and young children	For duration of illness
Viral hemorrhagic infections (Ebola, Lassa, Marburg)	For duration of illness
Zoster (chickenpox, disseminated zoster, or localized zoster in immunodeficient patients)	Until all lesions are crusted

ESSENTIAL STEPS
- Situate the patient in a private room with private toilet and an anteroom, if possible.
- Two patients with the same infection may share a room, if necessary.
- Put a "contact precautions" sign on the door to notify anyone entering the room and a sign on the chart to notify other departments that may come in contact with the patient. Check your facility's policy to determine proper signage.
- Wash your hands before entering and after leaving the patient's room and after removing gloves.
- Place laboratory specimens in impervious, labeled containers, and send them to the laboratory at once.

■ Attach completed requisition slips to the outside of the container.

■ Tell visitors to wear gloves and a gown while visiting the patient and to wash their hands after removing the gown and gloves.

■ Place all items that have come in contact with the patient in a single impervious bag, and arrange for their disposal or disinfection and sterilization.

■ Limit the patient's movement from the room.

■ If the patient must be moved, cover draining wounds with clean dressings.

■ Notify the receiving department of the patient's isolation precautions so they can be maintained and the patient returned to the room promptly.

SPECIAL CONSIDERATIONS

■ It's essential to clean and disinfect equipment between patients.

■ Dedicate certain reusable equipment (thermometer, stethoscope, blood pressure cuff) for the patient on contact precautions to reduce the risk of transmitting the infection to other patients.

■ Change your gloves during patient care as indicated by the procedure or task.

■ Wash your hands after removing gloves and before putting on new gloves.

■ Reinforce the need for contact precautions and review isolation procedures with the patient and his family.

■ Reinforce that all visitors must wear gloves and a gown while visiting, and that they should wash their hands when leaving after removing the gown and gloves.

■ Remind the patient that he isn't to leave his room and that only he should use his toilet.

■ Reinforce teaching regarding infection control techniques, such as good hand washing, with the patient and his family.

COMPLICATIONS

None known.

DOCUMENTATION

■ Record the need for contact precautions, as indicated by your facility.

■ Document the dates that contact precautions were started and maintained.

■ Note the patient's tolerance of procedure.

■ Document reinforced teaching with the patient and his family.

■ Record the date contact precautions were stopped.

Droplet precautions

Droplet precautions prevent the spread of infectious diseases transmitted when nasal or oral secretions from an infected patient come in contact with mucous membranes of another person. Droplets of moisture, which arise from coughing or sneezing, are heavy and usually fall to the ground within 3′ (0.9 m). The organisms contained in droplets don't become airborne or suspended in air. (See *Diseases requiring droplet precautions.*) Effective droplet precautions require a private room—not necessarily one with negative airpressure—and the door doesn't need to be closed. Persons with direct contact or within 3′ of patient should wear a surgical mask covering the nose and mouth.

LIFE STAGES When handling infants or young children who require droplet precautions, you may also need to wear gloves and a gown to prevent soiling clothing with nasal and oral secretions.

CONTRAINDICATIONS
None known.

EQUIPMENT
Masks ● gowns (if necessary) ● gloves ● plastic bags ● isolation door card ● thermometer ● stethoscope ● blood pressure cuff

PREPARATION OF EQUIPMENT
■ Keep supplies outside patient's room in a cart or anteroom.

ESSENTIAL STEPS
■ Put patient in a private room with private toilet facilities and an anteroom, if possible.
■ Put a "droplet precautions" sign on the door to notify anyone entering the room and on the chart to notify other departments that may come in contact with the patient. Refer to the facility's policy to determine the proper signage.
■ Wash your hands before entering the room, after leaving the room, and during patient care as indicated.
■ Pick up your mask by the top strings, adjust it around your nose and mouth, and tie the strings for a comfortable fit.
■ If the mask has a flexible metal nose strip, adjust it to fit firmly but comfortably.
■ Tape an impervious plastic bag to the patient's bedside so he can properly dispose of facial tissues.

Diseases requiring droplet precautions

DISEASE	PRECAUTIONARY PERIOD
Adenovirus infection in infants and young children	For duration of illness
Diphtheria (pharyngeal)	Until antibiotic therapy ends and two cultures taken at least 24 hours apart are negative
Influenza	For duration of illness
Invasive *Haemophilus influenzae* type B disease, including meningitis, pneumonia, and sepsis	Until 24 hours after start of effective therapy
Invasive *Neisseria meningitidis* disease, including meningitis, pneumonia, epiglottiditis, and sepsis	Until 24 hours after start of effective therapy
Mumps	For 9 days after start of swelling
Mycoplasma pneumoniae infection	For duration of illness
Parvovirus B19	In immunodeficient patients with chronic disease, for duration of hospitalization. In patients with transient aplastic crisis or red-cell crisis, for 7 days.
Pertussis	Until 5 days after start of effective therapy
Pneumonic plague	Until 72 hours after start of effective therapy
Rubella (German measles)	Until 7 days after start of rash
Severe acute respiratory syndrome	For duration of illness (airborne precautions preferred)
Streptococcal pharyngitis, pneumonia, or scarlet fever in infants and young children	Until 24 hours after start of effective therapy
Viral hemorrhagic infections (Ebola, Lassa, Marburg)	For duration of illness

- Make sure all visitors wear masks when within 3′ of the patient and, if necessary, gowns and gloves.
- Make sure the patient wears a surgical mask over his nose and mouth when he leaves the room.
- Notify receiving department of isolation precautions so they can be maintained and the patient returned to his room promptly.
- Two patients with the same infection may share a room, if necessary.

SPECIAL CONSIDERATIONS
- Before removing your mask, remove gloves (if worn), and wash your hands.
- Untie the strings and dispose of your mask, handling it by the strings only.
- Reinforce the explanation of droplet precaution procedures with the patient and his family.
- Reinforce that the patient should cover his nose and mouth with facial tissue while coughing or sneezing.
- Review hygiene techniques, such as good hand washing, with the patient and his family.

COMPLICATIONS
None known.

DOCUMENTATION
- Record the need for droplet precautions, as indicated by your facility.
- Document the dates droplet precautions were started and maintained.
- Describe the patient's tolerance of precautions.
- Record reinforced patient and family teaching.
- Document the date droplet precautions were stopped.

3

I.V. THERAPY AND MEDICATION ADMINISTRATION

Most hospitalized patients receive some form of I.V. therapy. Although you may not be called on to insert every type of I.V. line, you'll be responsible for administering I.V. therapy, maintaining the lines, and preventing complications throughout therapy. This chapter explains the administration methods and primary uses of I.V. therapy.

Drug infusion through a secondary I.V. line

A secondary I.V. line is a complete I.V. set—container, tubing, and microdrip or macrodrip system—connected to the lower Y-port (secondary port) of a primary line instead of being connected directly to an I.V. catheter or needle. The secondary line permits continuous or intermittent drug infusion and titration while the primary line maintains a constant total infusion rate.

Most drugs can be piggybacked with a needleless system through a "piggyback port." I.V. pumps may be used to maintain constant infusion rates, allow accurate titration of dosages, and maintain venous access. (See *Assembling a piggyback set*, page 42.)

For an intermittent infusion, the primary line has a piggyback port with a backcheck valve that stops primary line flow during drug infusion and returns to primary line flow after infusion. A volume-control set can also be used with an intermittent infusion line.

Assembling a piggyback set

A piggyback set is useful for intermittent drug infusion. To work properly, the secondary set's container must be positioned higher than the primary set's container.

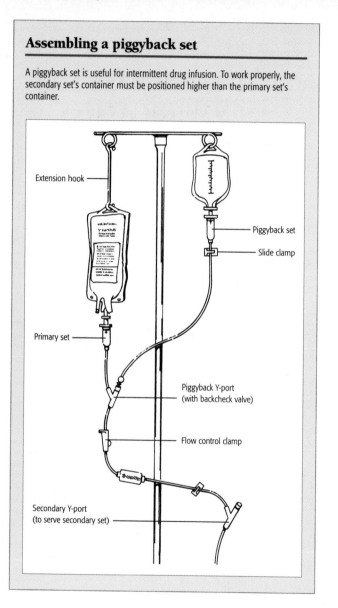

CONTRAINDICATIONS
None known.

EQUIPMENT
Patient's medication record and chart ● I.V. medication ● I.V. solution ● administration set with secondary injection port ● needleless adapter ● alcohol pads ● 1″ adhesive tape ● time tape ● labels ● infusion pump ● extension hook and appropriate solution for intermittent piggyback infusion ● normal saline solution for infusion with incompatible solutions (optional)

PREPARATION OF EQUIPMENT
■ Inspect the I.V. container for cracks, leaks, and contamination.
■ Verify expiration date.
■ Use an I.V. set with a secondary injection port if the drug is to be given regularly.

ESSENTIAL STEPS
■ Verify the order on the patient's drug record by checking it against the physician's order.
■ Wash your hands and put on gloves, if needed.
■ Confirm the patient's identity using two patient identifiers, such as the patient's name and identification number.
■ If your facility uses a bar code scanner, scan your ID badge, the patient's ID bracelet, and the drug's bar code.
■ Check drug compatibility with primary solution.

RED FLAG If the drug is incompatible with the primary I.V. solution, replace the primary solution with normal saline solution and flush the line before starting the drug infusion.

■ As needed, add the drug to the secondary I.V. solution; remove any seals from the secondary container and wipe the main port with an alcohol pad.
■ Inject the drug into the port and gently agitate to mix the drug thoroughly.
■ Properly label the I.V. mixture.
■ Insert the administration set spike and attach the needleless system.
■ Open the flow clamp, prime the line, and then close the flow clamp.
■ If the drug is in a container that's ready to hang on an I.V. pole, disengage the diluent so it mixes with the drug. Agitate the container, making sure the solution is well mixed. Insert the administration spike, prime the tubing, and hang the set.

- If required, remove the primary I.V. solution and put in a sterile plug until it's rehung. This maintains the sterility and prevents use of the incompatible solution before the line is flushed with normal saline solution.
- Hang the secondary set's container and wipe the injection port of the primary line with an alcohol pad.
- Insert the needleless adapter from the secondary line into the injection port, and secure it to the primary line.
- To run the secondary set's container by itself, lower the primary set's container with an extension hook.
- To run both containers simultaneously, place them at the same height.
- Open the clamp and adjust drip rate.
- For continuous infusion, set the secondary solution to desired drip rate; adjust the primary solution to the desired total infusion rate.
- For intermittent infusion, adjust the primary drip rate, as required, on completion of the secondary solution.
- If secondary solution tubing is being reused, close the clamp on the tubing and follow facility policy.
- Remove the needleless adapter and replace it with a new one, or leave the system secured in the injection port and label it with the time of first use.
- Leave the empty container in place until you replace it with a new dose of drug at the prescribed time.
- If tubing won't be reused, discard it appropriately.

SPECIAL CONSIDERATIONS

- If facility policy allows, use a pump for drug infusion.
- Put a time tape on the secondary container.
- When reusing secondary tubing, change it according to facility policy (at least every 72 hours).
- Inspect the injection port for leakage with each use and change, if needed.
- Don't piggyback a secondary I.V. line to a total parenteral nutrition line because of risk of contamination. TPN should always be infused using a sterile port. Check facility policy for any exceptions.
- Reinforce the explanation regarding the particular I.V. therapy and its purpose to the patient.
- Remind the patient what drug is being given.
- Reinforce that the patient should inform you of adverse reactions or problems.

COMPLICATIONS

The patient may develop an adverse reaction to the infused drug. Repeated punctures of the secondary injection port can damage the seal, which can cause leakage or contamination.

DOCUMENTATION

- Record the amount and type of drug and the I.V. solution on intake and output and drug records.
- Note the date, duration, and rate of infusion.
- Note the patient's response.

Intermittent infusion device insertion

Filled with normal saline solution to prevent clotting, an intermittent infusion device, also known as a *saline lock*, maintains venous access in patients receiving I.V. drugs regularly or intermittently but not continuously. This system keeps the access device sterile and prevents blood from leaking from the open end. Much like the administration set injection port, the intermittent injection cap is self-sealing after the needleless injector is removed. The device minimizes the risk of fluid overload and electrolyte imbalance better than a slow infusion with an I.V. to keep the vein open. It increases patient comfort and mobility, reduces anxiety, and may allow for multiple blood sample collection without repeated venipuncture.

CONTRAINDICATIONS

None known.

EQUIPMENT

Intermittent infusion device ● needleless system device ● normal saline solution ● tourniquet ● alcohol pad or other approved antimicrobial solution (such as chlorhexidine) ● venipuncture equipment ● transparent semipermeable dressing ● tape ● prefilled saline cartridges (available for use in a syringe cartridge holder) ● 1 ml of dilute heparin solution in a 3-ml syringe (optional)

ESSENTIAL STEPS

- Wash your hands.
- Confirm the patient's identity using two patient identifiers, such as the patient's name and identification number.
- Reinforce the explanation of the procedure.
- Remove the set from its packaging, wipe the port with an alcohol pad, and inject normal saline solution to fill or prime the tubing

BEST PRACTICE

Applying a tourniquet

To safely apply a tourniquet, follow these steps.

1. Place the tourniquet (preferably latex-free) under the patient's arm, about 6″ (15.2 cm) above the venipuncture site. Position the arm on the middle of the tourniquet.

2. Bring the ends of the tourniquet together, placing one on top of the other.

3. Holding one end on top of the other, lift and stretch the tourniquet and tuck the top tail under the bottom tail. Don't allow the tourniquet to loosen.

4. Tie the tourniquet smoothly and snugly; be careful not to pinch the patient's skin or pull his arm hair.

NO LONGER THAN 2 MINUTES

Leave the tourniquet in place for no longer than 2 minutes. If you can't find a suitable vein and prepare the venipuncture site in this amount of time, release the tourniquet for a few minutes. Then reapply it and continue the procedure. You may need to apply the tourniquet, find the vein, remove the tourniquet, prepare the site, and then reapply the tourniquet for the venipuncture.

AS FLAT AS POSSIBLE

Keep the tourniquet as flat as possible. It should be snug but not uncomfortably tight. If it's too tight, it will impede arterial as well as venous blood flow. Check the patient's radial pulse. If you can't feel it, the tourniquet is too tight and must be loosened. Also loosen and reapply the tourniquet if the patient complains of severe tightness.

and needleless system. This removes air, preventing an air embolus.

■ Select a venipuncture site.

■ Put on gloves and necessary personal protective equipment.

■ Apply a tourniquet 2″ (5.1 cm) proximal to the chosen area. (See *Applying a tourniquet*.)

■ Using a vigorous side-to-side motion, clean the venipuncture site with alcohol or other antimicrobial solution such as chlorhexidine; allow the solution to dry.

■ Perform the venipuncture, and ensure correct needle placement in the vein.

■ Release the tourniquet.

■ Tape the set in place.

■ Loop the tubing, if applicable, so the injection port is accessible.

■ Flush the catheter with normal saline solution. Some facilities use a dilute heparin flush solution; follow facility policy and procedure.

RED FLAG Be sure to remove the tourniquet before flushing the catheter.

■ Apply a transparent semipermeable dressing.
■ Write the time and date and your initials on the dressing label, and place it on the dressing.
■ Remove and discard your gloves.
■ Inject normal saline solution every 8 to 24 hours, or according to facility policy, to maintain the patency of the intermittent infusion device.
■ Inject normal saline solution slowly to prevent stinging.

SPECIAL CONSIDERATIONS
■ When accessing an intermittent infusion device, stabilize it to prevent dislodging from the vein.
■ If the patient feels burning during the injection of normal saline solution, stop the injection, check cannula placement, and monitor the site for infiltration or infection.
■ If the cannula is in the vein, inject the normal saline solution slower to minimize irritation. If the needle isn't in the vein, remove the needle and discard it; then perform the procedure again.
■ Change the intermittent infusion device every 48 to 72 hours, according to facility policy, using a new venipuncture site.
■ A transparent semipermeable dressing allows a greater patient freedom and better observation of the injection site.
■ If the physician orders an I.V. infusion stopped and an intermittent infusion device inserted, convert the existing line by disconnecting the I.V. tubing and inserting a male adapter plug into the device. (See *Converting an I.V. line to an intermittent infusion device,* page 48.)
■ Most health care facilities require the use of luer-lock systems on all infusion cannulas and lines.

COMPLICATIONS
Intermittent infusion devices have the same potential complications as a peripheral I.V. line.

DOCUMENTATION
■ Record the date and time of insertion and the name of the person who inserted the device.
■ Note the type, brand, and gauge of needle.
■ Document the length of cannula.
■ Record the anatomic location of insertion site.

Converting an I.V. line to an intermittent infusion device

The male adapter plug shown below allows you to convert an existing I.V. line into an intermittent infusion device. To make the conversion, follow these steps.

1. Prime the male adapter plug with saline solution.
2. Clamp the I.V. tubing and remove the administration set from the catheter or needle hub.
3. Insert a male adapter plug and twist it into place.
4. Flush the access with the remaining solution to prevent occlusion.

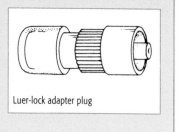

Luer-lock adapter plug

■ Note the patient's tolerance of the procedure.
■ Document the date and time of each saline flush.

I.V. infusion pumps

Various types of electronic I.V. infusion pumps are available to help regulate the flow of I.V. solutions or drugs, improving the safety and accuracy of drug and fluid administration. Pumps have various detectors and alarms that automatically signal completion of infusion, the presence of air in the line, low battery power, and occlusion or the inability to deliver the infusion at set rate. These devices may sound or flash an alarm, shut off, or switch to a keep-open rate.

CONTRAINDICATIONS
None known.

EQUIPMENT
Pump ● I.V. pole ● I.V. solution ● sterile pump administration set ● adhesive tape

PREPARATION OF EQUIPMENT
■ Attach the pump to the I.V. pole.
■ Insert the administration set spike into the I.V. container, and fill the drip chamber to prevent air bubbles from entering the tubing.

- Follow manufacturer's instructions for priming and placing the I.V. tubing.
- Flush all the air out of the tubing before connecting it to the patient to lower the risk of an air embolism.
- To avoid fluid overload, clamp the tubing whenever the pump door is open.

ESSENTIAL STEPS

- Confirm the physician's order and verify the patient's identity using two patient identifiers, such as the patient's name and identification number.
- Position the pump on the same side of the bed as the I.V. or anticipated venipuncture site, to avoid crossing I.V. lines over the patient.
- If necessary, perform the venipuncture.
- Plug in the machine and attach its tubing to the catheter hub.
- Depending on the machine, turn it on and press the start button.
- Set appropriate dials on the front panel to desired infusion rate and volume to be infused.
- Flush the I.V. with normal saline, if necessary, monitor for infiltration, and monitor the accuracy of the infusion rate.
- Tape all connections.
- Turn on alarm switches.
- Reinforce the explanation of the alarm system to the patient to prevent anxiety when the alarm is activated.

SPECIAL CONSIDERATIONS

- Monitor the pump and patient frequently to ensure correct operation, proper infusion rate, to detect infiltration, and to observe for such complications as infection and air embolism.
- Keep the pump plugged in when possible to ensure that the battery is fully charged at all times.
- If electrical power fails, the pump automatically switches to battery power.
- Change the tubing and cassette every 72 hours, or according to facility policy.
- Reinforce the explanation of the use and purpose of the pump or controller to the patient and his family. If necessary, repeat the demonstration of how the device works.

COMPLICATIONS

Complications are the same as those associated with peripheral lines such as infiltration, phlebitis, or occlusion.

DOCUMENTATION
■ Document the I.V. infusion.
■ Record the use of a pump on the I.V. record and in your notes.

I.V. infusion rate calculation and manual control

Calculated from a physician's orders, infusion rate is expressed as total volume of I.V. solution infused over a prescribed interval or as total volume given in milliliters per hour.

Many devices are used to regulate flow of I.V. solution, including clamps, the flow regulator (or rate minder), and the infusion pump. When regulated by a clamp, the infusion rate is usually measured in drops per minute; when regulated by an infusion pump, in milliliters per hour.

Infusion rate regulators can be set to deliver a desired amount of solution, also in milliliters per hour; they're less accurate than infusion pumps and are most reliable when used with inactive adult patients. The infusion rate can be monitored by using a time tape, which indicates the prescribed solution level at hourly intervals.

CONTRAINDICATIONS
None known.

EQUIPMENT
I.V. administration set with clamp ● 1″ paper or adhesive tape (or premarked time tape) ● infusion pump and pump administration set ● watch with second hand ● drip rate chart, as needed ● pen

PREPARATION OF EQUIPMENT
■ A standard macrodrip set delivers 10, 15, or 20 drops/ml, depending on the manufacturer, and a microdrip set delivers 60 drops/ml. (See *Calculating infusion rates.*)
■ An adapter can convert a macrodrip set to a microdrip set.

ESSENTIAL STEPS
■ Infusion rate requires close monitoring and correction; factors such as venous spasm, venous pressure changes, patient movement or manipulation of the clamp, and bent or kinked tubing can cause rate to vary. (See *Managing I.V. infusion rate deviations,* pages 52 and 53.)

(Text continues on page 54.)

Calculating infusion rates

When calculating the infusion rate (drops per minute) of I.V. solutions, remember that the number of drops required to deliver 1 ml varies with the type of administration set used and its manufacturer:

● Administration sets are of two types—macrodrip (the standard type) and microdrip. Macrodrip delivers 10, 15, or 20 drops/ml, depending on the manufacturer; microdrip usually delivers 60 drops/ml (see illustrations).

● Manufacturers calibrate their devices differently, so be sure to look for the "drop factor"—expressed in drops per milliliter, or gtt/ml—in the packaging that accompanies the set you're using. (This packaging also has crucial information about such things as special infusions and blood transfusions.)

When you know your device's drop factor, use the following formula to calculate specific infusion rates:

$$\frac{\text{Volume of infusion (in milliliters)}}{\text{Time of infusion (in minutes)}} \times$$

Drop factor (in drops per milliliter) =

Infusion rate (in drops per minute)

After you calculate the infusion rate for the set you're using, remove your watch or position your wrist so you can look at your watch and the drops at the same time. Next, adjust the clamp to achieve the ordered infusion rate and count the drops for 1 full minute. Readjust the clamp as necessary and count the drops for another minute. Keep adjusting the clamp and counting the drops until you have the correct rate.

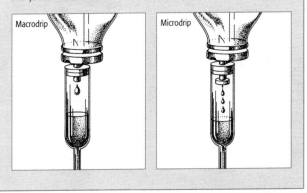

Macrodrip

Microdrip

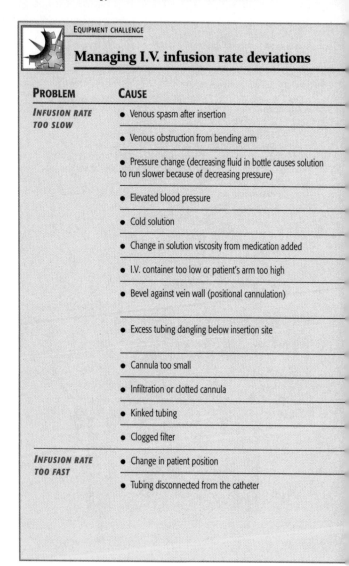

EQUIPMENT CHALLENGE

Managing I.V. infusion rate deviations

PROBLEM	CAUSE
INFUSION RATE TOO SLOW	● Venous spasm after insertion
	● Venous obstruction from bending arm
	● Pressure change (decreasing fluid in bottle causes solution to run slower because of decreasing pressure)
	● Elevated blood pressure
	● Cold solution
	● Change in solution viscosity from medication added
	● I.V. container too low or patient's arm too high
	● Bevel against vein wall (positional cannulation)
	● Excess tubing dangling below insertion site
	● Cannula too small
	● Infiltration or clotted cannula
	● Kinked tubing
	● Clogged filter
INFUSION RATE TOO FAST	● Change in patient position
	● Tubing disconnected from the catheter

INTERVENTION

- Apply warm soaks over site.

- Secure with an arm board if necessary.

- Readjust the infusion rate.

- Readjust the infusion rate. Use an infusion pump to ensure correct infusion rate.

- Allow the solution to warm to room temperature before hanging.

- Readjust the infusion rate.

- Hang the container higher or remind the patient to keep his arm below heart level.

- Withdraw the needle slightly, or place a folded 2″ × 2″ gauze pad over or under the catheter hub to change the angle.

- Replace the tubing with a shorter piece or tape the excess tubing to the I.V. pole below the flow clamp (make sure the tubing isn't kinked).

- Remove the cannula in use and insert a larger-bore cannula or use an infusion pump.

- Remove the cannula in use and insert a new cannula.

- Check the tubing over its entire length and unkink it.

- Remove the filter and replace it with a new one.

- Administer the I.V. solution with an infusion pump to ensure the correct infusion rate.

- Replace tubing, insert firmly into cannula hub, and tape at connection site. If replacement tubing isn't readily available, insert a male adapter plug into I.V. cannula hub until new tubing can be connected.
- The cannula may clot if tubing is disconnected for a length of time; if cannula is clotted, remove and insert a new one.

Calculating and setting the drip rate
■ Follow the steps in calculating infusion rates to determine the proper drip rate, or use your unit's drip rate chart.
■ After calculating the desired drip rate, hold your watch next to the drip chamber of the I.V. set and time the drops.
■ Release the clamp to the approximate drip rate, then count drops for 1 minute, to account for flow irregularities.
■ Adjust clamp as needed and count drops for another minute. Continue to adjust clamp and count drops until correct rate is achieved.

Making a time tape
■ Calculate the number of milliliters to be infused per hour. Place a piece of tape vertically on the container alongside the volume-increment markers.
■ Starting at the current solution level, move down the number of milliliters to be infused in 1 hour; mark the time and a horizontal line on the tape at this level. Mark 1-hour intervals until you get to the bottom of the container.
■ Check the infusion rate every 15 minutes until stable, then recheck every hour, or according to facility policy, and adjust as needed.
■ With each check, inspect the I.V. site for complications and monitor the patient's response to therapy.

SPECIAL CONSIDERATIONS
■ If the infusion rate slows significantly, a slight rate increase may be needed. If the rate must be increased more than 30%, consult the physician.
■ Use an I.V. pump to avoid infusion rate inaccuracies when possible. A pump is always used to infuse solutions using central venous access devices.
■ Large-volume solution containers have about 10% more fluid than the amount indicated on the bag, to allow for tubing purges.

COMPLICATIONS
An infusion rate that is too slow may cause insufficient intake of fluids, drugs, and nutrients. An rate infusion that is too rapid may cause circulatory overload, which could lead to heart failure, pulmonary edema, and adverse drug effects.

DOCUMENTATION
■ Record the original infusion rate when setting up a peripheral line.

■ If you adjust the rate, record the change, the date, and the time.
■ Document the amount of I.V. fluid infused on the intake and output sheet.

I.V. therapy preparation

Appropriate equipment selection and preparation are essential for
accurate delivery of I.V. solution; selection depends on rate and type
of infusion desired and on type of solution container used.

A macrodrip set delivers a large amount of solution quickly. A
microdrip set delivers a smaller amount of solution; it is used for
pediatric patients and adults requiring small or closely regulated
amounts of solution.

Tubing with secondary injection ports permits separate or simultaneous infusion of two or more solutions. Tubing with a piggyback port and backcheck valve permits intermittent infusion of a
secondary solution and return to infusion of the primary solution
when the secondary solution is completed. Vented I.V. tubing is
used for solutions in nonvented bottles. Nonvented tubing is used
for solutions in bags or vented bottles.

CONTRAINDICATIONS
None known.

EQUIPMENT
I.V. solution ● alcohol pad ● I.V. administration set ● in-line filter, if
needed ● I.V. pole ● drug and label, if needed

PREPARATION OF EQUIPMENT
■ Verify the type, volume, and expiration date of I.V. solution and
  the physician's order.
■ For solutions in a glass bottle, inspect for chips and cracks; for
  solutions in a plastic bag, squeeze the bag to detect leaks.
■ Examine the I.V. solution for particles, abnormal discoloration, or
  cloudiness.

> ▶ *RED FLAG If particles, abnormal discoloration, or cloudiness are*
> *present, discard the solution and notify the pharmacy and the*
> *physician.*

■ If ordered, add the drug to the solution and place a completed
  drug-added label on the container.
■ Remove the administration set from its box and check it for
  cracks, holes, and missing clamps.

ESSENTIAL STEPS

■ Confirm the physician's order and correctly identify the patient using two patient identifiers, such as the patient's name and identification number.

■ Wash your hands.

■ Slide the flow clamp of the administration set tubing down to the drip chamber or injection port, and close the clamp.

Preparing a bag

■ Place the bag on a flat, stable surface.

■ Remove the protective cap or tear the tab from the tubing insertion port.

■ Remove the protective cap from the administration set spike.

■ Holding the port firmly with one hand, insert the spike with your other hand.

■ Hang the bag on the I.V. pole, and squeeze the drip chamber until it's half full.

Preparing a nonvented bottle

■ Remove the bottle's metal cap and inner disk, if present.

■ Place the bottle on a stable surface and wipe the rubber stopper with an alcohol pad.

■ Open the vent port on the administration set, if necessary.

■ Remove the protective cap from the vented administration set spike, and push the spike through the center of the bottle's rubber stopper.

⚡ **RED FLAG** *Avoid twisting or angling the spike to prevent pieces of the stopper from breaking off and falling into the solution.*

■ Invert the bottle. If its vacuum is intact, you'll hear a hissing sound and see air bubbles rise (this may not occur if you've already added drug).

■ If the vacuum isn't intact, discard the bottle and begin again.

■ Hang the bottle on the I.V. pole, and squeeze the drip chamber until it's half full.

Preparing a vented bottle

■ Remove the bottle's metal cap and latex diaphragm to release the vacuum. If the vacuum isn't intact (except after drug has been added), discard the bottle and begin again.

■ Place the bottle on a stable surface and wipe the rubber stopper with an alcohol pad.

- Remove the protective cap from the nonvented administration set spike and push the spike through the insertion port next to the air vent tube opening.
- Hang the bottle on the I.V. pole, and squeeze the drip chamber until it's half full.

Priming the I.V. tubing

- If necessary, attach a filter to the opposite end of the I.V. tubing, and follow manufacturer's instructions for filling and priming.
- Purge the tubing before attaching the filter to avoid forcing air into the filter and clogging filter channels.
- Most filters are positioned with the distal end of the tubing facing upward so the solution completely wets the filter membrane and all air bubbles are eliminated from the line.
- If you aren't using a filter, aim the distal end of the tubing over a wastebasket or sink and slowly open the flow clamp. Be careful not to contaminate the distal end of the tubing by touching it to the surface of the wastebasket or sink.
- Some distal tube coverings allow the solution to flow without having to remove the protective cover.
- Leave the clamp open until the I.V. solution flows through the entire length of tubing to release trapped air bubbles and force out all the air.
- Invert all Y-ports and backcheck valves and tap them, if needed, to fill them with solution.
- After priming the tubing, replace the sterile cap on the end of the tubing and close the clamp.
- Loop the tubing over the I.V. pole.
- Label the container with patient's name and room number, date and time, container number, ordered rate and duration of infusion, your initials, and the date and time the solution expires.

SPECIAL CONSIDERATIONS

- Always use sterile technique when preparing I.V. solutions.
- If necessary, you can use vented I.V. tubing with a vented bottle. If doing so, don't remove the latex diaphragm. Instead, insert the spike into the larger indentation in the diaphragm.
- Change I.V. tubing every 72 hours, according to facility policy, or more frequently if you suspect contamination.
- Change the filter according to the manufacturer's recommendations, or sooner if it becomes clogged.
- Before starting I.V. therapy, correctly identify the patient, reinforce that the patient will have a plastic catheter or that a needle

will be placed in his vein. Remind him how long the catheter or needle will need to stay in place.

■ Remind the patient that the physician will decide what fluids he needs.

■ Reinforce that the patient receiving I.V. fluid may feel cold at first but the feeling will subside.

■ Remind the patient to report discomfort.

■ Reinforce restrictions.

COMPLICATIONS
None known.

DOCUMENTATION
■ Document how the patient was prepared for the procedure.

■ Document the time and date the solution was initiated, when the bag or bottle was changed, the amount of solution infused, and the rate of infusion in your notes and on the intake and output sheet.

■ Document the site used for I.V. access and describe the condition of the site.

Peripheral I.V. catheter insertion and removal

Peripheral I.V. therapy is ordered whenever venous access is needed; for example, when a patient requires surgery or emergency care. You may also use peripheral I.V. therapy to maintain hydration or provide fluid resuscitation, restore fluid and electrolyte balance, and for medication administration.

The device and site selection depend on type of solution used; the frequency and duration of infusion; the patency and location of accessible veins; the patient's age, size, and condition; and, if possible, the patient's preference. Preferred venipuncture sites are the cephalic and basilic veins in the lower arm and veins in the dorsum of the hand.

RED FLAG Be careful when placing an I.V. in the dorsum of the hand. Be sure the patient can bend his wrist with restricting I.V. flow if this site is selected. Patients with an I.V. in the back of the hand often have trouble walking with a walker because of wrist flexion.

If possible, choose a vein in the nondominant arm or hand. Antecubital veins can be used if no other venous access is available.

CONTRAINDICATIONS
■ Sclerotic vein
■ Edematous or impaired arm or hand
■ Postmastectomy or lymph node dissection
■ Burns
■ Arteriovenous fistula

EQUIPMENT
Alcohol pads or an approved antimicrobial solution, such as chlorhexidine ● gloves and necessary personal protective equipment ● tourniquet (latex-free) ● I.V. access devices ● I.V. solution with attached and primed administration set ● I.V. pole ● transparent semipermeable dressing ● 1″ hypoallergenic tape ● arm board and roller gauze (optional)

PREPARATION OF EQUIPMENT
■ Make sure that the I.V. solution container label includes the patient's name and another patient identifier, type of solution, time and date of preparation, preparer's name, ordered infusion rate, and expiration date.
■ Select an appropriate-gauge device.
■ If using a winged infusion set, connect the adapter to the administration set and unclamp the line until fluid flows from the open end of the needle cover.
■ Close the clamp and place the needle on a sterile surface.
■ If using a catheter device, open its package to allow easy access.

ESSENTIAL STEPS
■ Hang the I.V. solution with primed administration set on the I.V. pole.
■ Verify the physician's order and confirm the patient's identity using two patient identifiers.
■ Wash your hands.
■ Put on personal protective equipment.
■ Reinforce the explanation of the procedure to the patient.

Selecting the site
■ If long-term therapy is anticipated, start with a vein at the most distal site so you can move proximally as needed for subsequent sites.
■ For infusion of an irritating medication, choose a large vein distal to any nearby joint.
■ Choose a vein that can accommodate the cannula.

- Place the patient in a comfortable, reclining position, leaving the arm in a dependent position to increase venous fill of the lower arms and hands.
- If the patient's skin is cold, warm it by rubbing his arm, covering it with warm packs, or submerging it in warm water for 5 to 10 minutes.

Applying the tourniquet

- Apply a tourniquet approximately 6″ (15.2 cm) above the intended venipuncture site.
- Leave the tourniquet in place no longer than 2 minutes.
- Monitor for a radial pulse. If it isn't present, release the tourniquet and reapply it with less tension to prevent arterial occlusion.
- Lightly palpate the vein with the index and middle fingers of your nondominant hand.
- Stretch the skin to anchor the vein. If the vein feels hard or rope-like, select another.
- If you've selected a vein in the arm or hand that's palpable but not sufficiently dilated, tell the patient to open and close his fist several times.

Preparing the site

- Put on gloves and personal protective equipment and, if necessary, clip the hair around the insertion site.
- Clean the site with a facility-approved antimicrobial solution. Use a vigorous side-to-side motion to remove flora that would otherwise be introduced into the vascular system with the venipuncture. Allow the solution to dry.
- Lightly press the skin with the thumb of your nondominant hand about 1½″ (3.8 cm) from the intended insertion site.
- If you're using a winged infusion device, hold the short edges of the wings (with the needle's bevel facing upward) between the thumb and forefinger of your dominant hand and squeeze the wings together.
- If you're using an over-the-needle cannula, grasp the plastic hub with your dominant hand, remove the cover, and examine the cannula tip. If the edge isn't smooth, discard and replace the device.
- Using the thumb of your nondominant hand, pull the skin taut below the puncture site to stabilize the vein.
- Tell the patient that you're about to insert the needle.
- Hold the needle bevel-side up and enter the skin directly over the vein at a 0- to 15-degree angle.

- Push the needle through the skin and into the vein in one motion.
- Check the flashback chamber behind the hub for a blood return.
- Level the insertion device slightly by lifting the tip of the device up to prevent puncturing the back wall of the vessel.

If you're using a winged infusion device:
- Advance the needle fully and hold it in place.
- Release the tourniquet and open the administration set and clamp slightly.
- Check for a free flow or an infiltration.

If you're using an over-the-needle cannula:
- Advance the device to at least half of its length to make sure that the cannula itself, not just the introducer needle, has entered the vein. You can also advance the cannula slightly following the flashback of blood to make sure the outer cannula has entered the vein.
- Remove the tourniquet.
- Grasp the cannula hub to hold it in the vein and withdraw the needle. As you withdraw it, press slightly on the catheter tip to prevent bleeding.
- Advance the cannula up to the hub or until you meet resistance.
- To advance the cannula while infusing I.V. solution, release the tourniquet and remove the inner needle.
- Using sterile technique, attach the I.V. tubing and begin the infusion.
- While stabilizing the vein with one hand, use the other to advance the catheter into the vein.
- Decrease the I.V. infusion rate when the catheter is advanced.
- To advance the cannula before starting the infusion, release the tourniquet, stabilize the vein and needle, and advance the catheter off the needle and further into the vein up to the hub.
- Remove the inner needle quickly using sterile technique; attach the I.V. tubing.

Dressing the site
- Clean the skin completely.
- Use a transparent semipermeable dressing to secure the device (see *How to apply a transparent semipermeable dressing,* page 62).
- Loop the I.V. tubing on the patient's limb, and secure the tubing with tape.
- Label the last piece of tape with the type, gauge of needle, and length of the cannula; date and time of insertion; and your initials.

BEST PRACTICE

How to apply a transparent semipermeable dressing

Here's how to apply a transparent semipermeable dressing, which allows for visual assessment of the catheter insertion site:

● Make sure the insertion site is clean and dry.
● Remove the dressing from the package and, using sterile technique, remove the protective seal. Avoid touching the sterile surface.
● Place the dressing directly over the insertion site and the hub, as shown. Don't cover the tubing. Also, don't stretch the dressing; doing so may cause itching.
● Tuck the dressing around and under the catheter hub to make the site occlusive to microorganisms.

GRASP, LIFT, STRETCH
To remove the dressing, grasp one corner, and then lift and stretch.

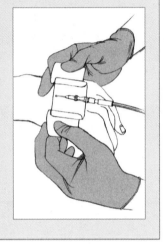

■ If needed, place an arm board under the joint and secure it with roller gauze or tape to provide stability. Make sure that the insertion site is visible and that the tape isn't constricting the patient's circulation. An armboard will prevent the patient from bending the joint and kinking the I.V. catheter, which will restrict the flow of I.V. fluids through the catheter.

Removing the I.V. line
■ Clamp the I.V. tubing to stop the flow of solution.
■ Gently remove the transparent dressing and tape from the skin.
■ Using sterile technique, open the gauze pad and adhesive bandage and place within reach.
■ Put on gloves and necessary personal protective equipment.
■ Hold the sterile gauze pad over the puncture site with one hand; use the other to withdraw the cannula slowly, keeping it parallel to the skin.

- Inspect the cannula tip; if it isn't smooth, assess the patient immediately, and notify the physician.
- Using the gauze pad, apply firm pressure over the puncture site for 1 to 2 minutes after removal, or until bleeding stops.
- Clean the site and apply the adhesive bandage or, if blood oozes, apply a pressure bandage.
- If drainage appears at the puncture site, swab the tip of the device across an agar plate or cut the tip into a sterile container using sterile scissors and send it to the laboratory to be cultured. Clean the area, apply a sterile dressing, and tell the physician that a sample was sent to the laboratory for culture.
- Remind the patient to restrict activity for about 10 minutes and to leave the dressing in place at least 1 hour.
- If tenderness persists at the site, apply warm packs and notify the physician.

SPECIAL CONSIDERATIONS

- If you fail to see flashback after the needle enters the vein, pull back slightly and rotate the device. If that doesn't work, remove the cannula and try again or proceed according to your facility's policy.
- Change a gauze or transparent dressing whenever you change the administration set (every 72 hours or according to facility policy).
- Rotate the I.V. site, at least every 72 hours or according to facility policy.
- Reinforce movement restrictions with the patient.
- Remind the patient to call the nurse if the infusion stops or an alarm goes off.

COMPLICATIONS

Complications of peripheral I.V. therapy can arise from the venous access device, the infusion, or the medication being administered and can be local or systemic. Local complications include infection, infiltration, phlebitis, cellulitis, catheter dislodgment, occlusion, vein irritation, hematoma, thrombophlebitis, and nerve, tendon, or ligament damage. Systemic complications include allergic reaction, sepsis, circulatory overload, and air embolism.

DOCUMENTATION

- Record the date and time of venipuncture.
- Record the name of person who inserted the device.
- Note the type, gauge, and length of the cannula.

- Document the anatomic location of the insertion site.
- Note the reason for site changes.
- Document the number of attempts at venipuncture.
- Record the type and infusion rate of the I.V. solution.
- Note the name and amount of drug in the solution and the expiration date.
- Document adverse reactions and actions taken.
- Record reinforced patient teaching.

Peripheral I.V. site maintenance

Routine maintenance of peripheral I.V. sites includes periodic site checks, site rotation, and changes of dressing, tubing, and solution. These measures help prevent complications, such as thrombophlebitis and infection, and should be performed according to your facility's policy and procedure.

CONTRAINDICATIONS
None known.

EQUIPMENT

For dressing changes
Gloves ● chlorhexidine or alcohol pads ● adhesive bandage ● transparent semipermeable dressing or sterile 2″ × 2″ gauze pad ● 1″ adhesive tape

For solution changes
Solution container (as ordered bag or bottle) ● alcohol pad

For tubing changes
I.V. administration set ● gloves ● sterile 2″ × 2″ gauze pad ● adhesive tape for labeling ● hemostat

For I.V. site changes
Alcohol pads or an approved antimicrobial solution such as chlorhexidine ● gloves ● tourniquet ● I.V. access device ● transparent semipermeable dressing ● 1″ hypoallergenic tape

PREPARATION OF EQUIPMENT
- Use a commercial dressing change kit if available.
- Keep I.V. equipment and dressings nearby.

■ If you're changing the solution and the tubing, attach and prime the I.V. administration set before entering the patient's room

ESSENTIAL STEPS
■ Wash your hands.
■ Wear gloves and necessary personal protective equipment.
■ Correctly identify the patient using two patient identifiers.
■ Reinforce the explanation of the procedure to the patient.

Changing the dressing
■ Remove the old dressing, open supply packages, and change gloves.
■ Hold the cannula in place with your nondominant hand.
■ Monitor the venipuncture site for signs of infection (redness and pain at the puncture site), infiltration (coolness, blanching, and edema at the site), and thrombophlebitis (redness, firmness, pain along the path of the vein, and edema).
■ If any of these signs are present, cover the area with a sterile $2'' \times 2''$ gauze pad and remove the catheter. Notify the physician. Apply a warm soak to an infiltrated site or a site with thrombophlebitis.
■ Apply pressure on the area until bleeding stops and apply an adhesive bandage.
■ Using fresh equipment and solution, start an I.V. in another appropriate site, preferably on the opposite extremity.
■ If the venipuncture site is intact, stabilize the cannula and carefully clean around the puncture site with a chlorhexidine swab or alcohol pad using vigorous side-to-side motion.
■ Allow the area to dry completely.
■ Cover the site with a transparent semipermeable dressing.
■ Place it over the insertion site to halfway up the hub of the cannula.

Changing the solution
■ Confirm the physician's orders and verify the patient's identity using two patient identifiers, such as the patient's name and identification number.
■ Wash your hands.
■ Inspect the new solution container for damage.
■ Check the solution for discoloration, turbidity, and particulates.
■ Note the date and time the solution was mixed and its expiration date.
■ Clamp the tubing when inverting it to prevent air from entering the tubing.

- Keep the drip chamber half full.
- If replacing a bag, remove the seal or tab from the new bag and remove the old bag from the pole.
- Remove spike, insert it into the new bag, and adjust the infusion rate.
- If you're replacing a bottle, remove the cap and seal from the new bottle and wipe the rubber port with an alcohol pad.
- Clamp the line, remove the spike from the old bottle, and insert the spike into the new bottle.
- Hang the new bottle and adjust the infusion rate.

Changing the tubing
- Reduce the I.V. infusion rate, remove the old spike from the container, and hang it on the I.V. pole.
- Place the cover of the new spike loosely over the old one.
- Keeping the old spike in an upright position above the patient's heart level, insert the new spike into the I.V. container.
- Prime the system.
- Hang the new I.V. container and primed set on the pole and grasp the new adapter in one hand.
- Stop the infusion rate in the old tubing.
- Put on gloves.
- Place a sterile gauze pad under the needle or cannula hub to create a sterile field.
- Press one of your fingers over the cannula to prevent bleeding.
- Gently disconnect the old tubing, being careful not to dislodge or move the I.V. device.
- Use a hemostat if needed to hold the hub securely while twisting the tubing to remove it, or use one hemostat on the venipuncture device and another on the hard plastic end of the tubing.
- Pull the hemostats in opposite directions. Don't clamp the hemostats shut; this may crack the tubing adapter or the venipuncture device.
- Remove the protective cap from the new tubing, and connect the new adapter to the cannula tip.
- Hold the hub securely to prevent dislodging the needle or cannula tip.
- Observe for blood backflow into the new tubing to verify that the needle or cannula is still in place.
- Adjust the clamp to maintain the appropriate infusion rate.
- Retape the cannula hub and I.V. tubing. Recheck the I.V. infusion rate because taping may alter it.
- Label the new tubing and container with the date and time.
- Label the solution container with a time strip.

SPECIAL CONSIDERATIONS

■ Check the prescribed I.V. infusion rate and physician's order before each solution change to prevent errors.
■ If you crack the adapter or hub (or if you accidentally dislodge the cannula from the vein), remove the cannula.
■ Apply pressure and an adhesive bandage to stop bleeding.
■ Perform a venipuncture at another site and restart the I.V.
■ Typically, I.V. dressings are changed when the device is changed, or when the dressing becomes wet, soiled, or nonocclusive.
■ I.V. tubing is changed every 72 hours or according to your facility's policy. The I.V. solution is changed every 24 hours or as needed.
■ The site should be assessed every 4 hours if a transparent semipermeable dressing is used. Otherwise, the site is assessed with every dressing change and should be rotated at least every 72 hours.

COMPLICATIONS

None known.

DOCUMENTATION

■ Note the time, date, rate, type of solution (and additives), and the expiration date on the I.V. flowchart.
■ Record dressing and tubing changes.
■ Document the appearance of the I.V. site in your notes.

Volume-control set

A volume-control set utilizes an I.V. line with a graduated chamber that delivers precise amounts of fluid and shuts off when the fluid is exhausted, preventing air from entering the I.V. line. The set may be used as a secondary line in adults for intermittent infusion of drugs. (See *Comparing I.V. administration sets,* pages 68 and 69.)

　RED FLAG A volume-control set is used as a primary line in children for continuous infusion of fluids or drug.

CONTRAINDICATIONS

None known

EQUIPMENT

Volume-control set ● I.V. pole (for setting up a primary I.V. line) ● I.V. solution ● needleless device ● alcohol pads ● drug in labeled syringe ● tape ● label

Comparing I.V. administration sets

I.V. administration sets come in three major types: basic (also called *primary*), add-a-line (also called *secondary*), and volume-control. The basic set is used to administer most I.V. solutions. An add-a-line set delivers an intermittent secondary infusion through one or more additional Y-sites or Y-ports. A volume-control set delivers small, precise amounts of solution. All three types come with vented or nonvented drip chambers.

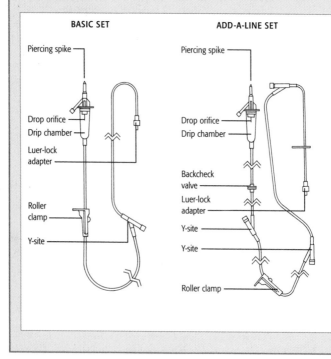

BASIC SET

- Piercing spike
- Drop orifice
- Drip chamber
- Luer-lock adapter
- Roller clamp
- Y-site

ADD-A-LINE SET

- Piercing spike
- Drop orifice
- Drip chamber
- Backcheck valve
- Luer-lock adapter
- Y-site
- Y-site
- Roller clamp

PREPARATION OF EQUIPMENT

- Various models of volume-control sets are available; each consists of a graduated fluid chamber (120 to 250 ml) with a spike and a filtered air line on top and administration tubing underneath.

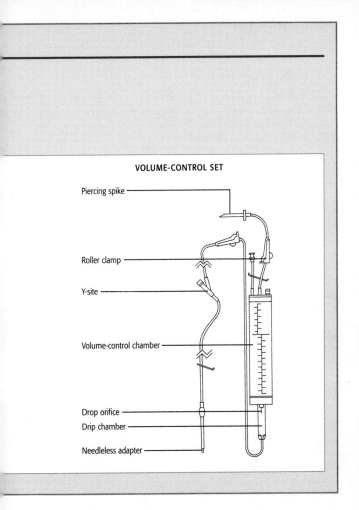

VOLUME-CONTROL SET

Piercing spike

Roller clamp

Y-site

Volume-control chamber

Drop orifice

Drip chamber

Needleless adapter

- Floating-valve sets have a valve at the bottom that closes when the chamber empties; membrane-filter sets have a rigid filter at the bottom that, when wet, prevents the passage of air.
- Ensure the sterility of all equipment and inspect it carefully to ensure the absence of flaws.
- Take the equipment to the patient's bedside.

ESSENTIAL STEPS

- Confirm the physician's order and correctly identify the patient using two patient identifiers, such as patient's name and identification number.
- Wash your hands.
- Reinforce the explanation of the procedure to the patient.
- If an I.V. line is already in place, check its insertion site for signs of infiltration and infection.
- Remove the volume-control set from its box and close all clamps.
- Remove the protective cap from the volume-control set spike, insert the spike into the I.V. solution container, and hang the container on the I.V. pole.
- Open the air vent clamp and close the upper slide clamp.
- Open the lower clamp on the I.V. tubing, slide it upward until it's slightly below the drip chamber, and close the clamp.
- If using a valve set, open the upper clamp until the fluid chamber fills with about 30 ml of solution; close the clamp and carefully squeeze the drip chamber until it's half full.
- If using a volume-control set with a membrane filter, open the upper clamp until the fluid chamber fills with about 30 ml of solution, then close the clamp.
- Open the lower clamp and squeeze the drip chamber flat with two fingers of your opposite hand.

  RED FLAG If you squeeze the drip chamber with the lower clamp closed, you'll damage the membrane filter.

- Keeping the drip chamber flat, close the lower clamp. Release the drip chamber so it fills halfway.
- Open the lower clamp, prime the tubing, and close the clamp.
- To use the set as a primary line, insert the distal end of the tubing into the catheter hub. To use as a secondary line, attach the needleless device to the adapter on the volume-control set.
- Wipe the Y-port of the primary tubing with an alcohol pad, and insert the needleless device and tape the connection.
- To add a drug, wipe the injection port on the volume-control set with an alcohol pad, and inject the drug.
- Label the chamber with the drug, dose, and date.

  RED FLAG Don't write directly on the chamber because the plastic absorbs ink.

- Open the upper clamp, fill the fluid chamber with the prescribed amount of solution, and close the clamp. Rotate the chamber to mix the drug.
- Turn off the primary solution (if present) or lower the drip rate to maintain an open line.

■ Open the lower clamp on the volume-control set, and adjust the drip rate as ordered.
■ After completion of the infusion, open the upper clamp and let 10 ml of I.V. solution flow into the chamber and through the tubing to flush them.
■ If using the volume-control set as a secondary I.V. line, close the lower clamp and reset the infusion rate of the primary line.
■ If using the set as a primary I.V. line, close the lower clamp, refill the chamber to the prescribed amount, and begin the infusion again.

SPECIAL CONSIDERATIONS
■ Always check compatibility of the drug and the I.V. solution.
■ If using a membrane-filter set, avoid giving suspensions through it.
■ If using a floating-valve set, the diaphragm may stick after repeated use. If it does, close the air vent and upper clamp, invert the drip chamber, and squeeze it. If the diaphragm opens, reopen the clamp and continue to use the set.
■ If the drip chamber of a floating-valve diaphragm set overfills, immediately close the upper clamp and air vent, invert the chamber, and squeeze excess fluid from the drip chamber back into the graduated fluid chamber.

COMPLICATIONS
None known.

DOCUMENTATION
■ Record the amount and type of drug you add to the volume-control set.
■ Note the amount of fluid used to dilute it and the amount of fluid infused on the intake and output record.
■ Document the date and time of infusion.

4

CARDIOVASCULAR CARE

Cardiovascular disorders affect millions of Americans each year. The responsibility of caring for patients with these disorders crosses nearly every area of nursing practice. With the continuing development of new drugs, diagnostic tests, and monitoring equipment, cardiovascular care is one of the most rapidly changing fields. Nurses face a constant challenge to keep up with the latest developments.

Automated external defibrillator

An automated external defibrillator (AED) is used for early defibrillation, which, along with cardiopulmonary resuscitation (CPR), is the most effective treatment for ventricular fibrillation and pulseless ventricular tachycardia. Some facilities require that an AED be present in every noncritical care unit. AEDs are also common in public places, such as shopping malls, sports stadiums, and airplanes. AEDs are increasingly being used to provide early defibrillation— even when no health care provider is present. The AED interprets the patient's cardiac rhythm and gives the operator step-by-step directions if defibrillation is needed. Most models are equipped with a microcomputer that senses and analyzes a patient's heart rhythm at the push of a button and will audibly or visually prompt the operator to deliver a shock. All AED models have the same basic function, but they offer different operating options; for example, some models have a simultaneous display of the patient's heart rhythm.

CONTRAINDICATIONS
- Don't use on a stable patient with a pulse.
- Don't use on a patient having a seizure.
- Don't use if the patient or his legal representative has made a legal documented request that the patient not be resuscitated.

■ Don't use if there's immediate danger to rescuers because of environment, patient's location, or patient's condition.

EQUIPMENT
AED ● two prepackaged electrodes ● gloves

PREPARATION OF EQUIPMENT
■ Make sure that the AED is plugged in and charging when not in use, per manufacturer's recommendations and your facility's policy.

ESSENTIAL STEPS
■ After determining that the patient is unresponsive, not breathing, and has no pulse, begin CPR. Follow basic life support guidelines.
■ Ask a colleague to bring the AED into the patient's room.
■ Open foil packets containing two electrode pads.
■ Turn on the power. Depending on the AED model, this may initiate voice prompts to guide the operator through subsequent steps. It may also prompt a self-test.
■ Put on gloves.
■ Expose the patient's chest.
■ Clip hair if needed and wipe sweat, oil, or lotion off the area where the electrode pads will be placed to ensure adequate skin contact.
■ Remove the plastic backing film from electrode pads and place them on the skin firmly and evenly in the following locations: one pad below the clavicle to the right of the sternum and one pad on the midaxillary line to the left of the left nipple; alternatively, place one pad anteriorly over the left apex and one pad in the infrascapular area posteriorly. (See *Automated external defibrillators*, page 74.)

RED FLAG Make sure there's good contact between each electrode and the skin so the AED can analyze the rhythm accurately and defibrillate properly. Don't place the electrode pads over bone. The energy released by the defibrillator can't pass through bone to reach the heart.

LIFE STAGES No AED is available for infants younger than age 1. If the victim is age 1 to 8 or weighs less than 55 lb (25 kg), use a pediatric electrode system.

■ Most AEDs signal readiness by a computerized voice that says, "Stand clear," or by emitting a series of loud beeps.

Automated external defibrillators

Automated external defibrillators (AEDs) vary with the manufacturer, but the basic components for each device are similar. This illustration shows a typical AED and proper electrode placement.

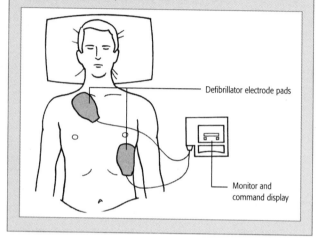

Defibrillator electrode pads

Monitor and command display

- If the AED is malfunctioning, it will convey the message "Do not use the AED. Remove and continue CPR." Obtain a functioning AED. Report the AED malfunction in accordance with your facility's procedure after the patient is stabilized.
- At this point the machine is ready to analyze the patient's heart rhythm.
- Press the ANALYZE button when prompted by the machine.

RED FLAG Be careful not to touch or move the patient while the AED is in analysis mode. If you get the message "Check electrodes," make sure the electrode pads are correctly placed and secured to the skin and the patient cable is securely attached; then press the ANALYZE button again.

- If a shock isn't needed, the AED will display "No shock indicated" and prompt you to "Check patient."
- If the patient needs a shock, the AED will display "Stand clear" and emit a beep that changes into a steady tone as it's charging.
- When the AED is fully charged and ready to deliver a shock, it will prompt you to press the SHOCK button. (Some fully automat-

ic AED models will give a warning and automatically deliver a shock within 15 seconds after analyzing patient's rhythm.)

■ Make sure no one is touching the patient or his bed, and call out "I'm clear, you're clear, everybody is clear."

■ Press the SHOCK button on the AED.

■ After the first shock, perform immediate CPR beginning with chest compressions for a total of five cycles (about 2 minutes) Then allow the AED to check the patient's rhythm.

■ If the patient is still in ventricular fibrillation, the AED will automatically begin recharging at a higher joule level to prepare for a second shock.

■ Repeat steps performed earlier before delivering another shock of 360 joules to the patient if a monophasic AED is being used.

■ The energy level delivered may be different when using a defibrillator that delivers biphasic shocks. Follow your facility's policy.

■ Continue CPR beginning with chest compressions until the code team leader arrives.

■ After the code, remove and transcribe the AED's computer memory module or tape, or prompt the AED to print a rhythm strip with code data.

■ Follow your facility's policy for analyzing and storing code data.

■ Monitor the patient's vital signs, cardiac rhythm, and physical findings closely.

■ Prepare the patient for transfer, if necessary.

SPECIAL CONSIDERATIONS

■ Be aware of your patient's code status as defined by physician's orders, patient's advance directives, or orders from the patient's legal representative.

■ Defibrillators vary by manufacturer. Familiarize yourself with your facility's equipment.

■ When an AED is used in an emergency situation, there often isn't time for a medical professional to provide an explanation to the family before the treatment. After the event, make sure the reason for the treatment is explained and provide emotional support to the patient and family.

■ If the victim is immersed in water, remove him from the water and quickly dry his chest before applying electrodes.

■ If the victim has an implanted pacemaker or internal cardiac defibrillator, place the electrodes at least 1″ (2.5 cm) to the side of the implanted device.

■ Remove transdermal medication patches on the chest and wipe the area clean if they are in a location where the electrodes will be placed.

COMPLICATIONS

The AED can cause accidental electric shock to care providers at the bedside. Some patients may suffer minor skin irritation or burns at the site of the electrodes because of the energy transferred, even with adequate conduction medium preapplied to the electrode pads.

DOCUMENTATION

- Provide a summary of actions to the code team leader and document the code on the appropriate form.
- Note the time the patient was found in cardiac arrest and whether the arrest was witnessed.
- Note when you started CPR, when you applied the AED, how many shocks were delivered, and the level of energy used for each shock.
- Note if and when the patient regained a pulse and document vital signs and physical findings.
- Note any care delivered after the cardiac arrest.
- Document any complications, per your facility's policy.

Cardiac monitoring

Cardiac monitoring is used in patients with conduction disturbances and those at risk for life-threatening arrhythmias. It allows continuous observation of the heart's electrical activity. Electrodes are placed on the patient's chest to transmit electrical signals that are converted into tracing of cardiac rhythm on an oscilloscope. The type of monitoring used may be hardwire or telemetry. With hardwire monitoring, the patient is connected to a bedside monitor on which the cardiac rhythm is displayed. It can also be transmitted for secondary display on a remote console. Telemetry uses a small, portable transmitter connected to an ambulatory patient that sends electrical signals to a display monitor at a remote location. Telemetry is useful for monitoring arrhythmias that occur during sleep, rest, exercise, or stress.

CONTRAINDICATIONS

None known.

EQUIPMENT

Cardiac monitor ● leadwires ● patient cable ● disposable pregelled electrodes (number of electrodes varies from three to five, depending on the type of monitoring system) ● alcohol pads ● 4″ × 4″ gauze pads ● paper for the rhythm strip printer ● scissors and washcloth (optional)

Additional telemetry monitoring equipment
Transmitter ● transmitter pouch ● new or fully charged telemetry battery pack ● leads ● electrodes

PREPARATION OF EQUIPMENT
■ Plug the cardiac monitor into an electrical outlet and turn it on.
■ If the monitor has the capability, enter the patient's identification data into the main monitoring unit so that his tracing is labeled with his name and room number.
■ Insert the cable into the appropriate socket in the monitor.
■ Connect the leadwires to the cable. In some systems, leadwires are permanently secured to the cable.
■ Each leadwire should indicate location for attachment to the patient: right arm (RA), left arm (LA), right leg (RL), left leg (LL), and chest (C). The indication should appear on the leadwire if it's permanently connected or at the connection of the leadwires and cable to the patient. They may also be color coded.
■ Connect an electrode to each leadwire, carefully checking that each leadwire is in its correct outlet.
■ For telemetry, put a new or fully charged battery in the transmitter.
■ Be sure to match the poles on the battery with polar markings on the transmitter case.
■ Test the battery's charge and test the unit to make sure it's operational by pressing the button at the top of the unit.
■ If the leadwires aren't permanently affixed to telemetry unit, attach them securely.
■ If the leadwires must be attached individually, be sure to connect each one to the correct outlet.

ESSENTIAL STEPS
Hardwire monitoring
■ Wash your hands.
■ Reinforce the explanation of the procedure to the patient, provide privacy, and expose his chest.
■ Determine electrode positions on the patient's chest based on the system and lead you're using. (See *Positioning monitoring leads*, pages 78 and 79.)

(Text continues on page 80.)

Positioning monitoring leads

This chart shows the correct electrode positions for the monitoring leads you'll use most often. For each lead, you'll see electrode placement for a five-leadwire system, a three-leadwire system, and a telemetry system.

In the two hardwire systems, the electrode positions for one lead may be identical to the electrode positions for another lead. In this case, you simply adjust the lead selector switch to display the lead you want. In some cases, you'll need to reposition the electrodes.

In the telemetry system, you can create the same lead with two electrodes that you can with three, simply by eliminating the ground electrode.

The illustrations below use these abbreviations: RA, right arm; LA, left arm; RL, right leg; LL, left leg; C, chest; and G, ground.

FIVE-LEADWIRE SYSTEM	THREE-LEADWIRE SYSTEM	TELEMETRY SYSTEM

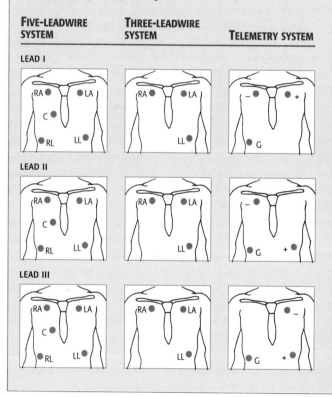

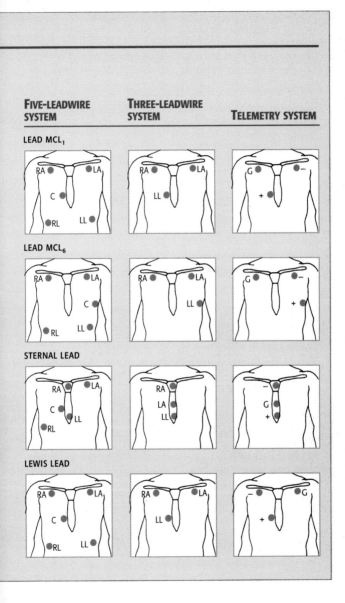

FIVE-LEADWIRE SYSTEM	THREE-LEADWIRE SYSTEM	TELEMETRY SYSTEM

LEAD MCL₁

LEAD MCL₆

STERNAL LEAD

LEWIS LEAD

■ If the leadwires and patient cable aren't permanently attached, verify that electrode placement corresponds to the label on the patient cable.

■ Clip the hair in an area about 4″ (10 cm) in diameter around each electrode site, if necessary.

■ Clean the area with an alcohol pad and dry completely to remove skin secretions or body lotion that may interfere with electrode function.

■ Gently abrade the dried area by rubbing it briskly with a dry washcloth or gauze until it reddens slightly to promote better electrical contact.

■ Remove backing from pregelled electrode.

■ Apply electrode to site and press firmly to ensure a tight seal.

■ Repeat process with remaining electrodes.

■ When all electrodes are in place, check for a tracing on the cardiac monitor.

■ Check the quality of the electrocardiogram. (See *Identifying cardiac monitor problems,* pages 82 to 85.)

■ To verify that the monitor is detecting each beat, compare the digital heart rate display with a minute-long count of the patient's apical heart rate.

■ If necessary, use "gain control" to adjust the size of the rhythm tracing and "position control" to adjust the waveform position on the recording paper.

■ Set upper and lower limits of heart rate alarm, based on the patient's heart rate, unit policy, and the physician's parameters.

■ Turn on the alarm and check the volume to make sure it's audible.

■ Make sure there's paper in the printer.

Telemetry monitoring

■ Make sure there's paper in the printer.

■ Wash your hands.

■ Reinforce the explanation of the procedure to the patient, provide privacy, and expose his chest.

■ Select the lead arrangement.

■ Attach an electrode to the end of each leadwire.

■ Remove the backing from one of the gelled electrodes.

■ Apply the electrode to appropriate site and press firmly to ensure a tight seal.

■ Repeat for each electrode.

- Place the transmitter in the pouch.
- Tie the pouch strings around the patient's neck and waist, making sure it fits snugly without causing discomfort.
- If no pouch is available, place the transmitter in the patient's bathrobe pocket.
- Check the patient's waveform for clarity, position, and size.
- Adjust the gain and baseline as needed.
- If necessary, ask the patient to remain resting or sitting in his room while you locate his telemetry monitor at the central station.
- Make sure the alarm is on and audible by temporarily setting the high limit lower than the patient's heart rate.
- Set upper and lower limits of heart rate alarm, based on the patient's heart rate, unit policy, and the physician's parameters.
- To obtain a rhythm strip, press the RECORD key at the central station.

SPECIAL CONSIDERATIONS

- Make sure all electrical equipment and outlets are grounded to avoid electric shock and interference (artifact).
- Avoid placing electrodes on bony prominences, hairy areas, areas where defibrillator pads will be placed, or areas for chest compression.
- If patient's skin is exceptionally oily, scaly, or diaphoretic, rub the electrode site with a dry 4″ × 4″ gauze pad before applying the electrode to reduce interference in tracing.
- Monitor skin integrity, and reposition the electrodes every 24 hours, or as needed, to prevent irritation or breakdown.
- If the patient is being monitored by telemetry, review with him how the transmitter works.
- Reinforce with the patient that the unit must be removed before bathing or showering, and remind him to tell the nurse before removing the unit.

COMPLICATIONS

The electrodes may cause skin irritation. Repositioning the electrodes every 24 hours (as necessary), or according to your facility's policy, will help prevent alterations in skin integrity.

DOCUMENTATION

- Record the date and time monitoring begins and which monitoring lead is used.

(Text continues on page 84.)

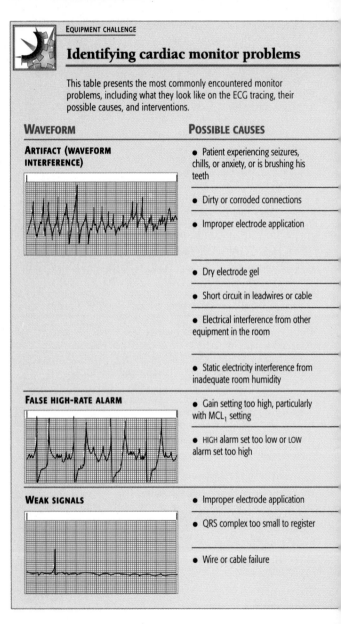

EQUIPMENT CHALLENGE

Identifying cardiac monitor problems

This table presents the most commonly encountered monitor problems, including what they look like on the ECG tracing, their possible causes, and interventions.

WAVEFORM	POSSIBLE CAUSES
ARTIFACT (WAVEFORM INTERFERENCE)	● Patient experiencing seizures, chills, or anxiety, or is brushing his teeth
	● Dirty or corroded connections
	● Improper electrode application
	● Dry electrode gel
	● Short circuit in leadwires or cable
	● Electrical interference from other equipment in the room
	● Static electricity interference from inadequate room humidity
FALSE HIGH-RATE ALARM	● Gain setting too high, particularly with MCL$_1$ setting
	● HIGH alarm set too low or LOW alarm set too high
WEAK SIGNALS	● Improper electrode application
	● QRS complex too small to register
	● Wire or cable failure

INTERVENTIONS

- If the patient is having a seizure, notify the physician and intervene as ordered.
- Keep the patient warm and encourage him to relax.

- Replace dirty or corroded wires.

- Check the electrodes and reapply them if needed. Clean the patient's skin well because skin oils, lotions, and dead skin cells inhibit conduction. Remove excess hair if it's preventing proper electrode-skin contact.

- Check the electrode gel. If the gel is dry, apply new electrodes.

- Replace broken equipment.

- Make sure all electrical equipment is attached to a common ground. Check all three-pronged plugs to ensure that none of the prongs are loose. Notify biomedical department. Unplug any equipment that doesn't need to be plugged in.

- Regulate room humidity to 40% if possible.

- Reset gain.

- Set alarm limits according to the patient's heart rate, physician's parameters, and your facility's policy.

- Reapply the electrodes.

- Reset gain so that the height of the complex is greater than 1 mV.
- Try monitoring the patient on another lead.

- Replace any faulty wires or cables.

(continued)

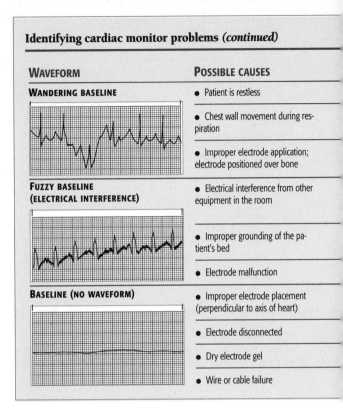

Identifying cardiac monitor problems (*continued*)

WAVEFORM	POSSIBLE CAUSES
WANDERING BASELINE	• Patient is restless
	• Chest wall movement during respiration
	• Improper electrode application; electrode positioned over bone
FUZZY BASELINE (ELECTRICAL INTERFERENCE)	• Electrical interference from other equipment in the room
	• Improper grounding of the patient's bed
	• Electrode malfunction
BASELINE (NO WAVEFORM)	• Improper electrode placement (perpendicular to axis of heart)
	• Electrode disconnected
	• Dry electrode gel
	• Wire or cable failure

■ Post a labeled rhythm strip in the patient's chart whenever there is a change in his condition.

■ Label the rhythm strip according to your facility's policy, usually with patient's name, date, and time (if it isn't preprinted on the strip). If it's preprinted, check the information for accuracy.

Defibrillation assistance

Defibrillation, the standard treatment for ventricular fibrillation or pulseless ventricular tachycardia, involves using electrode paddles to direct an electric current through the patient's heart. The current

INTERVENTIONS

- Encourage the patient to relax.

- Make sure that tension on the cable isn't pulling the electrode away from the patient's body.

- Reposition improperly placed electrodes.

- Make sure that all electrical equipment is attached to a common ground.
- Check all three-pronged plugs to make sure none of the prongs are loose.
- Unplug any equipment that doesn't have to be plugged in.

- Make sure that the bed ground is attached to the room's common ground.

- Replace the electrodes.

- Reposition improperly placed electrodes.

- Check if the electrodes are disconnected.

- Check the electrode gel. If the gel is dry, apply new electrodes.

- Replace any faulty wires or cables.

causes the myocardium to depolarize, which encourages the sinoatrial node to resume control of the heart's electrical activity. This current may be delivered by a monophasic or biphasic defibrillator. The electrode paddles delivering current may be placed on the patient's chest or, during or following cardiac surgery, directly on the myocardium. Because ventricular fibrillation leads to death if not corrected, the success of defibrillation depends on early recognition and quick treatment of arrhythmias.

CONTRAINDICATIONS
None known.

EQUIPMENT

Defibrillator (monophasic or biphasic) ● external paddles or internal paddles (sterilized for cardiac surgery) ● conductive medium pads or gel ● electrocardiogram (ECG) monitor with recorder ● oxygen therapy equipment ● handheld resuscitation bag ● intubation equipment ● emergency pacing equipment ● emergency cardiac drugs

PREPARATION OF EQUIPMENT

▪ The defibrillator should be ready for use at all times.
▪ When not in use, it should be plugged in, charged, maintained, and checked according to the manufacturer's recommendations and your facility's policy.

ESSENTIAL STEPS

▪ Determine that the patient is unresponsive and call for help.
▪ Check airway, breathing, and circulation and perform cardiopulmonary resuscitation (CPR) according to basic life support guidelines until the defibrillator, emergency equipment, and code team arrive.
▪ Designate one member of the health care team to document the events of the treatment.
▪ If the defibrillator has "quick-look" capability, the paddles will be placed on the patient's chest to quickly view the cardiac rhythm.
▪ Connect the cardiac monitoring leads of the defibrillator to the patient and check for a rhythm.
▪ The patient's chest will be exposed and conductive pads will be applied to paddle placement positions, or conductive gel will be applied to the paddles.
▪ For anterolateral placement, one paddle will be placed to the right of the upper sternum, just below the right clavicle, and the other over the fifth or sixth intercostal space at the left anterior axillary line.
▪ For anteroposterior placement, the anterior paddle will be positioned directly over the heart at the precordium to the left of the lower sternal border.
▪ The flat posterior paddle will be placed under the patient's body beneath the heart and immediately below the scapulae (not under the vertebral column).
▪ The defibrillator will be turned on and, if external defibrillation will be performed, the energy level will be set at 360 joules for an adult patient when using a monophasic defibrillator.

LIFE STAGES *When a pediatric patient is being defibrillated, make sure the appropriate paddles are used and proper joule level is selected.*

RED FLAG *When defibrillation is performed directly on the myocardium, make sure the appropriate paddles are used and proper joule level is selected.*

■ Clinically appropriate energy levels must be determined for a biphasic defibrillator.

■ The paddles will be charged by pressing the CHARGE buttons, located either on the machine or on the paddles themselves.

■ The physician or advanced cardiac life support (ACLS)–trained registered nurse who will be defibrillating will place the paddles over the conductive pads and press firmly against the patient's chest, using 25 pounds of pressure.

■ Observe the patient's cardiac rhythm.

■ If it's determined that the patient remains in ventricular fibrillation or pulseless ventricular tachycardia, the physician or ACLS-trained registered nurse discharging the paddles will tell all personnel to stand clear of the patient and the bed by stating "I'm clear, you're clear, we're all clear," and will then discharge the current by pressing both paddle CHARGE buttons simultaneously.

RED FLAG *Make sure that none of the monitor cables or electrodes are touching the defibrillator paddles.*

■ After the shock is delivered, CPR should be resumed, beginning with chest compressions for five cycles.

■ Observe the patient's cardiac rhythm and monitor the patient's pulse.

■ Prepare for a second defibrillation, if necessary.

■ The energy level on the defibrillator will be reset to 360 joules, or the biphasic energy equivalent.

■ The physician or ACLS-trained registered nurse defibrillating will announce that he's preparing to defibrillate, and will repeat the procedure.

■ Resume CPR, give supplemental oxygen, and assist as appropriate. Drugs such as epinephrine are given.

■ The code team should consider possible causes for failure of the patient's rhythm to convert, such as acidosis or hypoxia.

■ If defibrillation restores a normal rhythm, monitor the patient's central and peripheral pulses and obtain a blood pressure reading, heart rate, and respiratory rate.

■ Monitor the patient's level of consciousness, cardiac rhythm, breath sounds, skin color, and urine output.

- Monitor arterial blood gas levels and obtain a 12-lead ECG.
- Provide supplemental oxygen and ventilation, as needed.
- Check the patient's chest for electrical burns and treat them, as ordered, with corticosteroid or lanolin-based creams.
- Prepare the patient for transfer, if necessary.

SPECIAL CONSIDERATIONS

- Defibrillators vary by manufacturer; familiarize yourself with your facility's equipment. Most defibrillators have the capability to convert to defibrillator pads in place of paddles.
- Defibrillator operation should be checked as per manufacturer's recommendations and your facility's policy.
- Defibrillation can be affected by several factors, including paddle size and placement, condition of the patient's myocardium, duration of the arrhythmia, chest resistance, and number of counter-shocks.
- There are precautions that need to be taken before defibrillation takes place. (See *Safety issues with defibrillation.*)
- Cardiac arrest should be managed by an ACLS team composed of a team leader and one or more team members.
- In emergency situations, there usually isn't time to educate the family before the procedure. When the event is over, provide emotional support to the patient and family and reinforce the rationale for the treatment.

COMPLICATIONS

Defibrillation can cause accidental electric shock to those providing care. The patient may suffer skin burns from the energy transferred during defibrillation.

DOCUMENTATION

- Document the procedure, including the patient's ECG rhythm both before and after defibrillation.
- Report the number of times defibrillation was performed and the number of joules used with each defibrillation.
- Note whether a pulse returned.
- Record the dosage, route, and time of drug administration.
- Report whether CPR was performed and how the airway was maintained.
- Document the patient's response to treatment and any complications.

Safety issues with defibrillation

Precautions must be taken when a physician or advanced cardiac life support-trained registered nurse is defibrillating a patient who is in contact with water or a patient with an implantable cardioverter-defibrillator (ICD), a pacemaker, or a transdermal medication patch.

DEFIBRILLATING A PATIENT WITH AN ICD OR PACEMAKER
The defibrillator paddles or pads shouldn't be placed directly over the implanted device. They should be at least 1″ (2.5 cm) away from the device.

DEFIBRILLATING A PATIENT WITH A TRANSDERMAL MEDICATION PATCH
The defibrillator paddles or pads shouldn't be placed directly on top of a transdermal medication patch, such as a nitroglycerin, nicotine, analgesic, or hormone replacement patch. The patch can block delivery of energy and cause a small burn to the skin. Remove the medication patch and wipe the area clean before defibrillation.

DEFIBRILLATING A PATIENT NEAR WATER
Water is a conductor of electricity and may provide a pathway for energy from the defibrillator to the rescuers treating the victim. Remove the patient from freestanding water and dry him off before defibrillation.

Electrocardiography

Electrocardiography (ECG) is a valuable diagnostic tool that measures the heart's electrical activity as waveforms. Impulses moving through the heart's conduction system create electric currents that can be monitored on the body's surface. Electrodes attached to the skin can detect these electric currents and transmit them to an instrument that produces a record (the electrocardiogram) of cardiac activity. ECG can be used to help diagnose myocardial ischemia and infarction, rhythm and conduction disturbances, chamber enlargement, electrolyte imbalances, and drug toxicity. ECG uses 10 electrodes to measure electrical potential from 12 different leads. This creates the standard ECG complex, called PQRST. (See *Reviewing electrocardiograph waveforms and components*.)

CONTRAINDICATIONS
None known.

Reviewing electrocardiograph waveforms and components

An electrocardiograph waveform has three basic components: the P wave, QRS complex, and T wave. These elements can be further divided into the PR interval, J point, ST segment, U wave, and QT interval.

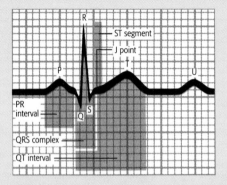

P WAVE AND PR INTERVAL
The P wave represents atrial depolarization. The PR interval represents the time it takes an impulse to travel from the atria through the atrioventricular nodes and bundle of His; it measures from the beginning of the P wave to the beginning of the QRS complex.

QRS COMPLEX
The QRS complex represents ventricular depolarization (the time it takes for the impulse to travel through the bundle branches to the Purkinje fibers).

The Q wave appears as the first negative deflection in the QRS complex; the R wave, as the first positive deflection. The S wave appears as the second negative deflection, or the first negative deflection after the R wave.

J POINT AND ST SEGMENT
The J point marks the end of the QRS complex and indicates the beginning of the ST segment. The ST segment represents part of ventricular repolarization.

T WAVE AND U WAVE
Usually following the same deflection pattern as the P wave, the T wave represents ventricular repolarization. The U wave follows the T wave, but isn't always seen.

QT INTERVAL
The QT interval represents ventricular depolarization and repolarization. It extends from the beginning of the QRS complex to the end of the T wave.

EQUIPMENT

ECG machine ● recording paper ● standard electrodes and gel or disposable pregelled electrodes ● alcohol pads ● 4″ × 4″ gauze pads ● clippers, marking pen (optional) ● scissors or shaving supplies (optional)

PREPARATION OF EQUIPMENT

■ Put the ECG machine close to the bed and plug it in, if necessary.
■ If the patient is already connected to a cardiac monitor, remove or temporarily move the electrodes to accommodate the precordial leads and minimize electrical interference on the ECG tracing.

 RED FLAG *Keep the patient away from electrical fixtures and power cords.*

ESSENTIAL STEPS

■ Verify the patient's identity using two patient identifiers, such as the patient's name and identification number.
■ Reinforce the explanation of the procedure, provide privacy, wash your hands, and wear nonsterile gloves.
■ Place the patient in the supine position with his arms at his sides. Ask him to remain as still as possible. If he can't tolerate lying flat, raise the head of the bed to semi-Fowler's position.
■ Expose the patient's arms and legs.
■ Have the patient relax his arms and legs to minimize muscle trembling, which can cause electrical interference and interfere with ECG tracing.
■ Make sure the patient's feet aren't touching the bed board.
■ Select flat, fleshy areas for the electrodes; avoid muscular and bony areas.
■ Clip or shave hair if needed.
■ Clean the skin with alcohol to enhance electrode contact; allow it to dry.
■ Peel off contact paper from the disposable electrodes and apply directly to the prepared site as recommended by the manufacturer.
■ To get the best leadwire connection, position disposable electrodes on the legs with the lead connection pointing superiorly.
■ Connect the limb leadwires to the electrodes.
■ Each leadwire is lettered and color-coded for easy identification: white goes to the right arm (RA), green to the right leg (RL), red to the left leg (LL), black to the left arm (LA), and brown to the chest (V_1 to V_6).

Positioning chest electrodes

To ensure accurate test results, position chest electrodes as follows:

V_1: Fourth intercostal space at right sternal border
V_2: Fourth intercostal space at left sternal border
V_3: Halfway between V_2 and V_4
V_4: Fifth intercostal space at left midclavicular line
V_5: Fifth intercostal space at left anterior axillary line (halfway between V_4 and V_6)
V_6: Fifth intercostal space at left midaxillary line, level with V_4

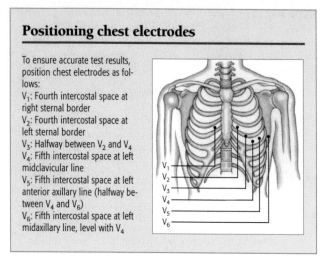

- Expose the patient's chest and put an electrode at each position. (See *Positioning chest electrodes*.)
- For a woman, place chest electrodes below the breast tissue; laterally displace breast tissue of a large-breasted woman.
- Set the paper speed selector to the standard 25 mm/second and the machine to full voltage. The machine will record a normal standardization mark.
- Enter appropriate patient identification data, as needed.
- If part of the waveform extends beyond the paper when recording, adjust the normal standardization to half-standardization and note the adjustment on the ECG strip.
- Ask the patient to relax, lie still, breathe normally, and refrain from talking.
- Press the AUTO or 12-LEAD button and observe tracing quality. The machine records all 12 leads automatically, recording three consecutive leads simultaneously. (Some machines have a display screen so you can preview waveforms before the machine records them on paper.)
- When the machine finishes recording the 12-lead ECG, remove the electrodes and clean the patient's skin.
- After disconnecting the leadwires from the electrodes, dispose of or clean the electrodes, as indicated.

■ Check the preprinted identification data or label the ECG with the patient's data.
■ Place the ECG printout in the chart according to your facility's policy.

SPECIAL CONSIDERATIONS
■ If the patient's respirations distort the recording, ask him to hold his breath briefly while you record the ECG.
■ If the patient has a pacemaker, contact the physician to determine if he would like to perform the ECG with a magnet.
■ Reinforce with the patient why the procedure is being done and that the test records the heart's electrical activity at certain intervals.
■ Remind the patient that the test doesn't hurt, won't cause electrical shock, and takes up to 10 minutes to perform.
■ Repeat the description of where the electrodes will be attached and remind the patient that the gel may feel cold.
■ Assist the patient to lie still and relax and remind him not to talk and to breathe normally.

COMPLICATIONS
Skin sensitivity reactions to the electrodes may occur.

DOCUMENTATION
■ Label the ECG recording with the patient's name, date and time, facility identification number, if it isn't printed by the machine. If it is printed by the machine, check that the data are correct.
■ Document the appropriate clinical information including head elevation if the patient was unable to lie flat for the procedure.
■ Record in your nursing notes the date and time of ECG.
■ Document the presence of a pacemaker and whether the physician used a magnet to turn it off.
■ Document significant patient responses.
■ Note the patient's tolerance of the procedure.

Permanent pacemaker

A permanent pacemaker is a self-contained heart pacing device implanted in a pocket beneath the patient's skin, designed to operate for 3 to 20 years. It consists of a pulse generator (which creates the electric impulse that stimulates the myocardium to contract and contains a battery), leads (insulated conductors that carry information from the electrodes to the pulse generator and electrical impulses from the generator to the heart muscle), and electrodes (which sense the heart's electrical activity). The device is inserted in the operating room or cardiac catheterization laboratory. It's used to treat irreversible heart conduction problems after a myocardial infarction, persistent bradyarrhythmias, second and third-degree heart block or slow ventricular rates, Stokes-Adams syndrome, Wolff-Parkinson-White syndrome, and sick sinus syndrome. A biventricular pacemaker may benefit a patient with heart failure. Pacing electrodes can be placed in the atria, ventricles, or in both chambers; most common pacing codes are VVI for single-chamber pacing and DDD for dual-chamber pacing.

CONTRAINDICATIONS
None known.

EQUIPMENT
Sphygmomanometer ● stethoscope ● electrocardiogram (ECG) monitor and strip-chart recorder ● povidone-iodine ointment ● sterile gauze dressing ● hypoallergenic tape ● I.V. line for emergency medications (optional)

PREPARATION OF EQUIPMENT
■ Verify the patient's identity using two patient identifiers, such as the patient's name and identification number.
■ Enter the patient's identification data into the cardiac monitor, if appropriate.
■ Make sure the monitor is placed on "paced mode" if it needs to be set manually.
■ Check to make sure the alarm is on and audible.

ESSENTIAL STEPS
■ Connect the patient to a cardiac monitor and observe for a rhythm.
■ Review the mode and base rate or lower and upper limits set on the pacemaker from the operative note in the chart.
■ Set the alarms to sound if the patient's heart rate falls below the base rate or lower limit or goes above the upper limit.
■ Continually monitor the patient's ECG and observe for pacing spikes. (See *Pacemaker spikes.*)
■ Observe the ECG tracing and monitor the patient's apical and radial pulse for 1 minute to make sure that they're equal and to ensure paced, and nonpaced beats, are profusing well.

Pacemaker spikes

Pacemaker impulses–the stimuli that travel from the pacemaker to the heart–are visible on an electrocardiogram tracing as spikes. Large or small pacemaker spikes appear above or below and perpendicular to the isoelectric line. This rhythm strip shows an atrial and a ventricular pacemaker spike.

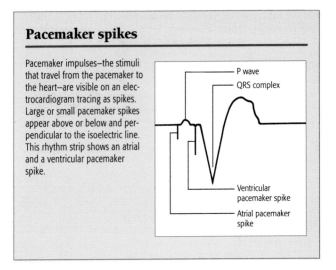

- P wave
- QRS complex
- Ventricular pacemaker spike
- Atrial pacemaker spike

- Monitor the patient for signs of pacemaker malfunction, including arrhythmias, syncope, hypotension, and a weak or thready pulse.
- Monitor the I.V. site if fluids are given.
- Check the dressing for bleeding according to your facility's policy.
- Prophylactic antibiotics may be ordered for up to 7 days after pacemaker implantation.
- Change the dressing and, after making sure the patient doesn't have an iodine allergy, apply povidone-iodine ointment at least once every 24 to 48 hours or according to your facility's policy.
- Monitor the surgical site for a hematoma or signs of infection.
- If the dressing becomes soiled or the site is exposed to air, change the dressing immediately.
- Check vital signs and level of consciousness (LOC) every 15 minutes for the first hour, every hour for the next 4 hours, every 4 hours for the next 48 hours, and then once every shift or according to facility policy.

LIFE STAGES Confused elderly patients with second-degree heart block won't show immediate improvement in LOC.

RED FLAG Report to the physician signs and symptoms of a perforated ventricle, with resultant cardiac tamponade: persistent hiccups, distant heart sounds, pulsus paradoxus, hypotension with *narrow pulse pressure, increased venous pressure, cyanosis, jugular vein distention, decreased urine output, pericardial friction rub, restlessness, or complaints of fullness in the chest.*

SPECIAL CONSIDERATIONS

■ The patient will be given an identification card that lists the pacemaker type and manufacturer, serial number, pacemaker rate setting, date implanted, and physician's name. Reinforce that the patient should carry the card on his person at all times and that he should keep a copy of it with his medical records.

■ Encourage the patient to review the literature about his pacemaker.

■ Reinforce the following teaching points with the patient:
  – The pacemaker augments the patient's natural heart rate.
  – The patient must tell his physicians, dentist, and other health care personnel that he has a pacemaker.
  – The patient should hold a cell phone up to his ear on the side opposite his pacemaker and move away from electrical equipment if he experiences light-headedness or dizziness. Moving away should restore normal pacemaker function.
  – The patient should avoid large magnetic fields, such as large motors or electrical substations.
  – The patient should avoid raising his arms above shoulder level for 24 hours and avoid heavy lifting or vigorous activity for 2 to 4 weeks after implantation. He should also avoid trauma to the site.
  – Tell the patient to clean his pacemaker site gently with soap and water during a shower or a bath and to leave the incision site exposed to the air.
  – The patient should inspect the skin around the incision daily; a slight bulge is normal, but he should call the physician if he feels discomfort or notices swelling, redness, discharge, or other problems.
  – The patient should check his pulse daily for 1 minute on the side of his neck, inside his elbow, or on the thumb side of his wrist. The pulse rate should be the same as his pacemaker rate or faster and he should notify the physician if he thinks his heart is beating too fast or too slow.
  – The patient should follow the medication schedule and understand the importance of keeping follow-up appointments with his physician.
  – Remind the patient to notify the physician if he experiences signs of pacemaker failure, such as palpitations, a fast heart

rate, a slow heart rate (5 to 10 beats less than the pacemaker's setting), dizziness, fainting, shortness of breath, hiccups, swollen ankles or feet, anxiety, forgetfulness, or confusion.

 RED FLAG *If the patient is pacemaker-dependent or is pacing continuously, place a transcutaneous pacemaker and transvenous pacemaker supplies at the bedside in case of a permanent pacemaker malfunction or failure.*

■ If the patient has a biventricular pacemaker, reinforce teaching and explain that a biventricular pacemaker has three leads instead of one or two; one lead is placed in the right atrium and the other two are placed in each of the ventricles, improving pumping efficiency.

COMPLICATIONS

The pulse generator, leads, electrodes, or incision may become infected. After surgical insertion the leads may be displaced from their intended position, which may cause arrhythmias and inappropriate sensing or pacing or failure to sense or pace. The ventricle may become perforated during the procedure or by the lead or electrode, causing bleeding and possible cardiac tamponade. The leads may also fracture or disconnect causing pacemaker malfunction.

DOCUMENTATION

■ Document the patient's status when he returns from the procedure (awake, alert, confused).

■ Record the patient's vital signs according to your facility's policy.

■ Label the patient's postoperative ECG or rhythm strip if the information isn't preprinted.

■ Record any symptoms the patient reports and any signs of pacemaker malfunction and include a rhythm strip printed at the same time.

■ Note the condition of the incision site and dates and times of dressing changes.

■ Record all medications given.

5

RESPIRATORY CARE

No matter where you work, you're sure to encounter patients with respiratory conditions. Such conditions may be acute or chronic and may have developed as a primary disorder or as a result of a cardiac or other disorder. Caring for the patient with a respiratory condition will challenge your nursing skills. To meet your care goals, you need to have a working knowledge of the therapies available to respiratory care patients.

Chest tube insertion and removal

The pleural space contains a thin layer of lubricating fluid that allows the visceral and parietal pleura to move without friction during respiration. Excess blood or bloody fluid (hemothorax), serous fluid (pleural effusion), air (pneumothorax), or air and fluid in the pleural space changes intrapleural pressure and may cause partial or complete lung collapse. Chest tube insertion allows air or fluid to be drained from the pleural space. It's usually performed by a physician with nurse assistance and it requires sterile technique. The insertion site varies depending on the patient's condition and the physician's judgment. After insertion, chest tubes are connected to a water-sealed thoracic drainage system, which removes air, fluid, or both from pleural space, prevents backflow, and promotes lung reexpansion.

CONTRAINDICATIONS
None known.

EQUIPMENT
Two pairs of sterile gloves • sterile drape • povidone-iodine solution • vial of 1% lidocaine • 10-ml syringe • alcohol pad • 22G 1″ needle • 25G ⅜″ needle • sterile scalpel (usually with #11 blade) • sterile forceps • two rubber-tipped clamps for each chest tube •

sterile 4″ × 4″ gauze pads ● two sterile 4″ × 4″ drain dressings (gauze pads with slit) ● 3″ or 4″ sturdy, elastic tape ● 1″ adhesive tape for connections ● chest tube of appropriate size (#16 to #20 French catheter for air or serous fluid; #28 to #40 French catheter for blood, pus, or thick fluid), with or without a trocar ● sterile Kelly clamp ● suture material (usually 2-0 silk with cutting needle) ● a separate and labeled thoracic drainage system for each chest tube: sterile drainage tubing, 6′ (1.8 m) long, and connector ● sterile Y-connector (for two chest tubes on the same side) ● petroleum gauze ● suction source, if necessary ● sterile water

PREPARATION OF EQUIPMENT

■ Check the expiration date on sterile packages and inspect for tears.
■ In a nonemergency situation, make sure the patient has signed a consent form.
■ Assemble equipment in the patient's room and set up the thoracic drainage system according to the manufacturer's directions.
■ Place the drainage system by the patient's bed below chest level to facilitate drainage.

ESSENTIAL STEPS

■ Verify the patient's identity using two patient identifiers, such as the patient's name and identification number.
■ Reinforce the explanation of the procedure to the patient, provide privacy, and wash your hands.
■ Confirm that the patient doesn't have allergies to iodine, tape, or latex.
■ Record baseline vital signs, including oxygen saturation level, and make sure a recent respiratory assessment is documented, including a description of baseline breath sounds.
■ Provide, or contact the registered nurse to provide, preprocedure analgesics as ordered.
■ Position the patient and tell him that he can best assist by lying as still as possible and by using relaxed breathing.
■ If the patient has pneumothorax, place him in high Fowler's, semi-Fowler's, or a supine position.
■ Before the procedure is started the team should take a "time out" to make sure the right procedure is being performed on the right patient at the right site.
■ The physician will insert the tube in the anterior chest at the midclavicular line in the second or third intercostal space.

- If the patient has hemothorax or pleural effusion, have him lean over the overbed table or straddle a chair with his arms dangling over the back.
- The physician will insert the tube in the sixth or seventh intercostal space at the midaxillary line.
- For either pneumothorax or hemothorax, the patient may lie on his unaffected side with his arms extended over his head.
- When you have positioned the patient properly, place the chest tube tray on the overbed table.
- Open the equipment using sterile technique.
- The physician will put on sterile gloves and prepare the insertion site by cleaning the area with povidone-iodine solution.
- Wipe the rubber stopper of the lidocaine vial with an alcohol pad.
- Invert the bottle and hold it for the physician to withdraw the anesthetic.
- After anesthetizing the site, the physician will make a small incision, insert the chest tube, and connect it to the thoracic drainage system.
- As the chest tube is inserted, reassure the patient and assist the physician as needed.
- The physician may secure the tube to the skin with sutures.
- Open the packages containing the petroleum gauze, 4″ × 4″ drain dressings and gauze pads, and put on sterile gloves.
- Place the petroleum gauze and two 4″ × 4″ drain dressings around the insertion site, one from the top and one from the bottom.
- Place several 4″ × 4″ gauze pads on top of the drain dressings.
- Tape the dressings using 3″ to 4″ elastic tape, covering them completely.
- Securely tape the chest tube to the patient's chest distal to the insertion site to prevent accidental dislodgment.
- Securely tape the junction of the chest tube and the drainage tube to prevent separation. Tape the junction securely, but make sure the tip of the drainage tube is visible within the clear chest tube so that if it disconnects it would be readily seen.
- Make sure the tubing remains level with the patient and there are no dependent loops or kinks.
- Immediately after the drainage system is connected, tell the patient to take a deep breath, hold it momentarily, and slowly exhale to assist drainage of the pleural space and lung reexpansion. The water in the drainage system should rise with inhalation and fall with exhalation.

■ The physician will order a portable chest X-ray to check the tube's position.

■ Check the patient's vital signs every 15 minutes for 1 hour, then as indicated or according to your facility's policy.

■ Monitor the patient's respiratory status at least every 4 hours after the procedure, or according to your facility's policy, to assess air exchange in the affected lung.

 RED FLAG *Diminished or absent breath sounds indicate that the patient's lung hasn't reexpanded.*

■ Monitor the amount, color, and consistency of the drainage. Record the drainage level in the drainage collection chamber and label it with the time and date.

SPECIAL CONSIDERATIONS

■ Clamping the chest tube isn't recommended because there's a risk of tension pneumothorax.

■ During patient transport, always keep the thoracic drainage system below his chest level.

■ Before transporting the patient who has a thoracic drainage system connected to suction, check with the physician to determine if the thoracic drainage system can be temporarily removed from suction.

■ Place rubber-tipped clamps at the bedside.

■ If drainage system cracks, or a tube disconnects, clamp the chest tube as close to the insertion site as possible.

 RED FLAG *No air or liquid can escape from the pleural space while the tube is clamped. Observe the patient closely for signs and symptoms of tension pneumothorax while the clamp is in place.*

■ As an alternative to clamping the tube, submerge the distal end in a container of normal saline solution, placed at a level that's lower than the patient's lung, to create a temporary water seal while you replace the drainage system. Follow your facility's policy.

■ The physician may order the tube to be clamped with large, smooth, rubber-tipped clamps for several hours before removal.

■ While the tube is clamped, monitor the patient for signs and symptoms of respiratory distress, an indication that air or fluid remains trapped in the pleural space.

■ The patient may require premedication with analgesics before the physician or advanced practitioner discontinues the chest tube.

■ Chest tubes are usually removed within 7 days to prevent infection. (See *Removing a chest tube,* page 102.)

Removing a chest tube

After a patient's lung has reexpanded, you may assist the physician or advanced practitioner in removing a chest tube. First, check the patient's vital signs and monitor his respiratory status. After reinforcing an explanation of the procedure, give an analgesic as ordered 30 minutes before tube removal. Have the registered nurse give I.V. analgesics. Then follow these steps:

● Place the patient in semi-Fowler's position or on his unaffected side.
● Place a linen-saver pad under the affected side.
● Put on clean gloves, remove chest tube dressings (being careful not to dislodge the chest tube), and discard soiled dressings.
● The physician or advanced practitioner will hold the chest tube in place with sterile forceps and cuts the suture anchoring the tube.
● The physician or advanced practitioner will make sure the chest tube is securely clamped, then he will instruct the patient to perform Valsalva's maneuver by exhaling fully and bearing down. Valsalva's maneuver effectively increases intrathoracic pressure.
● The physician or advanced practitioner will hold an airtight dressing, usually petroleum gauze, so he can cover the insertion site immediately after removing the tube.
● After the tube is removed and the site covered, secure the dressing with elastic tape. Cover the dressing completely to make it as airtight as possible.
● Dispose of the chest tube, soiled gloves, and equipment according to your facility's policy.
● Check the patient's vital signs, including oxygen saturation level, as ordered, and monitor depth and quality of respirations and breath sounds. Monitor carefully for signs and symptoms of pneumothorax, subcutaneous emphysema, or infection.

■ The patient may experience discomfort while the tube is in place and may require analgesics.
■ Reinforce teaching about the chest tube; remind the patient to call for assistance when getting in and out of bed so that the tube doesn't accidentally dislodge or disconnect.

RED FLAG If the chest tube comes out, leave the petroleum gauze in place and cover site immediately with 4″ × 4″ gauze pads and tape in place. Stay with the patient and monitor his vital signs every 10 minutes. Look for signs and symptoms of tension pneumothorax (hypotension, distended jugular veins, absent breath sounds, tracheal shift, hypoxemia, weak and rapid pulse, dyspnea, tachypnea, diaphoresis, chest pain). Have another staff member notify the physician and gather equipment needed to reinsert the tube.

COMPLICATIONS

Tension pneumothorax may result from excessive accumulation of air, drainage, or both, and eventually may exert pressure on the heart and aorta causing a precipitous fall in cardiac output. Bleeding is usually suspected if there is 200 ml or more of drainage from the tube in 1 hour. Subcutaneous emphysema or crepitus occurs when air leaks into the subcutaneous tissue surrounding the insertion site. Infection at the incision site or infection due to the presence of the drain can also occur.

DOCUMENTATION

- Document the date and time of chest tube insertion and the name of the physician who inserted it.
- Note a description of the insertion site and the color, consistency, and amount of drainage from the tube.
- Document the amount of output on the intake and output record.
- Indicate the drainage system used and the type and amount of suction applied, in appropriate.
- Report the presence of drainage and bubbling.
- Record the patient's vital signs.
- Note respiratory system findings.
- Note the time of the postprocedure chest X-ray.

Endotracheal tube care

Proper endotracheal (ET) tube care, which is important to ensure airway patency, includes monitoring airway status, maintaining proper cuff pressure, suctioning or repositioning the tube, and oral hygiene measures. The tube should be moved frequently from one side of the mouth to the other to prevent pressure ulcers.

CONTRAINDICATIONS

None known; however, patients with do-not-resuscitate orders aren't usually intubated.

EQUIPMENT
For maintaining the airway

Stethoscope ● suction equipment ● gloves ● handheld resuscitation bag with the appropriate adapter ● pulse oximeter

For repositioning the ET tube
10-ml syringe ● compound benzoin tincture ● stethoscope ● adhesive, hypoallergenic tape, or Velcro tube holder ● suction equipment ● sedative or 2% lidocaine ● gloves ● handheld resuscitation bag with mask in case of accidental extubation ● pulse oximeter ● 4″ × 4″ gauze

For removing the ET tube
10-ml syringe ● suction equipment ● supplemental oxygen source with mask ● cool-mist, large-volume nebulizer ● handheld resuscitation bag with mask or nasal cannula ● gloves ● equipment for reintubation ● pulse oximeter

PREPARATION OF EQUIPMENT
- Wash you hands before all procedures.
- Assemble equipment at the bedside.
- To assist the physician or respiratory therapist to reposition the ET tube, set up suction equipment using sterile technique.
- While the ET tube is being removed, set up suction and supplemental oxygen equipment and have equipment for emergency reintubation ready.

ESSENTIAL STEPS
- Reinforce the explanation of the procedure even if the patient doesn't seem alert.
- Provide privacy.
- Wear personal protective equipment when necessary.
- Put on gloves.

Maintaining airway patency
- Monitor the patient's respiratory status, observing for any sign of respiratory distress.
- If you detect an obstructed airway, determine the cause and treat it accordingly.
- If you suspect the patient is biting on the ET tube or to prevent him from biting, place an oral airway along the side of the ET tube and tape it in place.
- Suction secretions if they obstruct the lumen of the tube.
- If the ET tube appears to have slipped from the trachea into the right mainstem bronchus, indicated by absent breath sounds over the left lung fields, the physician will order a chest X-ray to verify tube placement and will reposition it if needed.

Assisting with repositioning the ET tube

■ Repositioning an ET tube requires two experienced, licensed personnel.

■ Before the tube is repositioned, suction the trachea through the ET tube to remove secretions, which can cause the patient to cough during the procedure.

■ To prevent aspiration during cuff deflation, suction the patient's pharynx to remove secretions that may have accumulated above the tube cuff.

■ Before the physician or respiratory therapist frees the tube, make sure the pilot balloon is out of the way and not in danger of being cut.

■ Locate a landmark or measure the distance from the patient's mouth to the top of the tube to get a reference point before the tube is moved.

■ When the tube is freed, deflate the cuff by attaching a 10-ml syringe to the pilot balloon port and aspirating air until you meet resistance and the pilot balloon deflates.

RED FLAG Deflate the cuff before the physician or respiratory therapist moves the ET tube because the cuff forms a seal within the trachea; movement of an inflated cuff can damage the tracheal wall and vocal cords.

■ Assist the physician or respiratory therapist to reposition the ET tube and to prevent accidental extubation during the procedure if the patient coughs. Note the new position landmarks or measure the length of the tube.

RED FLAG To prevent traumatic manipulation of the tube, make sure that the ET tube is held as the tube is carefully untaped or the Velcro tube holder is unfastened and as it's repositioned.

■ To reinflate the cuff, the physician or respiratory therapist will have the patient inhale and will slowly inflate the cuff using a 10-ml syringe attached to the pilot balloon port.

■ As the physician or respiratory therapist does this, he will use his stethoscope to auscultate the patient's neck to determine the presence of an air leak.

■ When air leakage stops, the physician or respiratory therapist will stop cuff inflation; while still auscultating the neck, he will aspirate a small amount of air until he detects a minimal air leak, indicating the cuff is inflated at the lowest possible pressure for an adequate seal.

■ If the patient is mechanically ventilated, a small amount of air will be aspirated to create a minimal air leak during the inspiratory phase because the positive pressure of the ventilator during inspiration will create a larger leak around the cuff.

- Note the amount of air required to achieve a minimal air leak.
- Measure cuff pressure and compare the reading with previous ones to prevent overinflation.
- The placement of the ET tube will be verified by auscultating both lung fields to verify breath sounds; auscultation over the epigastric area will confirm that the ET tube wasn't positioned in the stomach. Carbon dioxide levels may also be monitored to verify placement, and a chest X-ray may be required.
- Assist with applying compound benzoin tincture to the patient's cheeks and securely retape the tube using one continuous piece of tape. To avoid taping the patient's hair, double-face the tape on the back of the neck or use a 4″ × 4″ gauze. Leave a small amount of tape at the end and fold it back onto itself to grasp when removing. The tube can also be secured with a Velcro tube holder (the preferred method to secure the tube).
- Make sure the patient is comfortable and the airway patent.
- Measure cuff pressure at least every 8 hours to avoid overinflation.

Assisting with removing the ET tube

- To prevent traumatic manipulation during the removal of an ET tube, assist the physician or respiratory therapist.
- Raise the head of the patient's bed to about 90 degrees.
- Suction the patient's nasopharynx and oropharynx to remove accumulated secretions and to help prevent aspiration when the cuff is deflated.
- Using a handheld resuscitation bag or the mechanical ventilator, give the patient several deep breaths through the ET tube to hyperinflate his lungs and increase his oxygen reserve.
- Attach a 10-ml syringe to the pilot balloon port and aspirate air until you meet resistance and the pilot balloon deflates.

RED FLAG If an air leak isn't detected around the deflated cuff, the physician won't proceed with extubation. Absence of an air leak can indicate marked tracheal edema, which can cause total airway obstruction if the ET tube is removed.

- If the proper leak is detected, the physician or respiratory therapist will untape or unfasten the ET tube while the assisting nurse stabilizes it.
- The physician or respiratory therapist will insert a sterile suction catheter through the ET tube and apply suction. To reduce the risk of laryngeal trauma, he will ask the patient to take a deep breath, open his mouth fully, and pretend to cry out.
- Simultaneously, the physician or respiratory therapist will remove the ET tube and suction catheter in one smooth, outward and

downward motion, following the natural curve of the patient's mouth.

> *RED FLAG Suctioning during extubation removes secretions retained at the end of the tube and prevents aspiration.*

■ Give the patient supplemental oxygen. For humidity, use a cool-mist, large-volume nebulizer to decrease airway irritation and laryngeal edema.

■ Encourage the patient to cough and breathe deeply.

■ Make sure the patient is comfortable and his airway is patent.

■ After extubation, monitor the patient's respiratory status frequently and be alert for stridor or other evidence of upper airway obstruction.

■ Monitor arterial blood gas levels and oxygen saturation results, if available.

■ Provide mouth care.

SPECIAL CONSIDERATIONS

■ The patient may require sedation or instillation of 2% lidocaine to numb the airway when repositioning an ET tube if he has sensitive airways.

■ After extubation following a lengthy intubation, keep reintubation supplies available for at least 12 hours until you're sure the patient can tolerate extubation.

■ A patient shouldn't be extubated unless someone skilled at intubation is available.

■ If you inadvertently cut the pilot balloon on the cuff, leave the tube in place and immediately call the physician to remove and replace the damaged tube.

■ Always keep a handheld resuscitation bag at the bedside of a patient with an ET tube, along with the appropriate adapter for the specific sized tube.

■ Reinforce why the ET tube is being repositioned, how it will be done, and that the patient will need to keep his head still during repositioning.

■ Reinforce the explanation of how the ET tube will be removed and what he can do to help.

■ Remind the patient that he will be monitored closely after extubation.

■ Remind the patient to expect a sore throat and temporary hoarseness.

■ Reinforce the need for coughing, deep breathing, incentive spirometer use, and supplemental oxygen.

COMPLICATIONS

Traumatic injury to the larynx or trachea can occur during an intubation, while the tube is in place (from the balloon), or during extubation. The vocal cords can become irritated or paralyzed, causing the patient to have a hoarse voice. Airway obstruction may occur from a mucus plug or clot, resulting in hypoxia and respiratory failure. Laryngospasm and tracheal edema are other possible complications of having an ET tube in place.

DOCUMENTATION

- Document the number of times the patient was suctioned, a description of the secretions removed, and the patient's tolerance of the procedure.
- Note the date, time, and reason for tube repositioning.
- Document the new tube position.
- Record skin integrity at the former site and at the new site.
- Note the total amount of air in the cuff after the procedure and the cuff pressure.
- Record the date and time of extubation.
- Note any complications, including presence or absence of stridor or other signs of upper airway edema, and subsequent therapy.
- Document the type and amount of supplemental oxygen given, oxygen saturation level, and arterial blood gas results, if performed.

Manual ventilation

Manual ventilation delivers oxygen through a handheld resuscitation bag attached to a face mask or endotracheal (ET) or tracheostomy tube. It allows for the delivery of oxygen or room air to the lungs of a patient who can't breathe adequately by himself. When used in an emergency, it maintains ventilation while a patient is apneic, in respiratory failure, disconnected temporarily from a mechanical ventilator, being transported, or being prepared to be suctioned. Oxygen administration with a resuscitation bag can help improve a compromised cardiopulmonary system.

CONTRAINDICATIONS

- If the chest doesn't rise with manual ventilation, reposition the head. If the chest still doesn't rise, suspect airway obstruction. Stop ventilation and follow basic life support guidelines for airway obstruction.

EQUIPMENT

Handheld resuscitation bag with the appropriate adapter, if necessary ● face mask ● oxygen source (wall unit or tank) ● oxygen tubing ● nipple adapter attached to oxygen flowmeter ● gloves ● goggles ● oxygen accumulator, ● oxygen saturation monitor positive end-expiratory pressure valve (optional) (see *Using a positive end-expiratory pressure valve*, page 110)

PREPARATION OF EQUIPMENT

■ Unless the patient is intubated or has a tracheostomy (use appropriate adapter), select a mask that fits snugly over the mouth and nose.

■ Attach the mask to the resuscitation bag and the resuscitation bag to the nipple adaptor on the oxygen source.

■ Turn on the oxygen and adjust the flow rate according to the patient's condition and the physician's order. For example, if the patient has a low partial pressure of arterial oxygen, he'll need a higher fraction of inspired oxygen (FIO_2).

■ To increase the concentration of inspired oxygen, you can add an oxygen accumulator (also called an *oxygen reservoir*). This device, which attaches to an adapter on the bottom of the bag, permits an FIO_2 of up to 100%.

■ Once the manual resuscitation bag is ready, and if time allows, set up suction equipment.

■ Attach the patient to an oxygen saturation monitor, if available.

ESSENTIAL STEPS

■ Put on gloves and other personal protective equipment.

■ Before using the handheld resuscitation bag, check the patient's upper airway for foreign objects.

■ Remove obstructions if present. This alone may restore spontaneous respirations. Also, foreign matter or secretions can obstruct the airway and impede resuscitation efforts.

■ Suction the patient to remove secretions that may obstruct the airway.

■ If necessary, an oropharyngeal or nasopharyngeal airway may be inserted to maintain airway patency.

■ If the patient has a tracheostomy or ET tube in place, suction him.

■ If appropriate, remove the bed's headboard and stand at the head of the bed so you can help keep the patient's neck extended and free up space at the side of the bed for other activities such as cardiopulmonary resuscitation.

Using a positive end-expiratory pressure valve

Add positive end-expiratory pressure (PEEP) to manual ventilation by attaching a PEEP valve to the resuscitation bag. This may improve oxygenation if the patient hasn't responded to an increased fraction of inspired oxygen levels. Always use a PEEP valve to manually ventilate a patient who has been receiving PEEP on the ventilator.

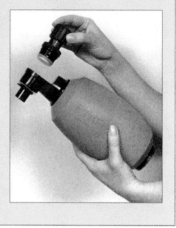

- Tilt the patient's head back, if not contraindicated, and pull his jaw forward to move the tongue away from the base of the pharynx and prevent obstruction of the airway. (See *How to use a handheld resuscitation bag.*)
- Using your nondominant hand, apply downward pressure to seal the mask against the patient's face.
- For an adult patient, use your dominant hand to compress the bag every 5 seconds to deliver about 1 L of air.

  LIFE STAGES *For infants and children, use a pediatric handheld resuscitation bag. Deliver 20 breaths/minute or one compression of the bag every 3 seconds and 250 to 500 cc of air with each bag compression.*

- Deliver manual ventilation with the patient's spontaneous inhalations, if present.
- Don't attempt to deliver a breath as the patient exhales.
- Observe the patient's chest to ensure that it rises and falls with each compression of the handheld resuscitation bag.
- If ventilation fails to occur, check the fit of the mask and the patency of the patient's airway; if necessary, reposition his head and ensure patency with an oral airway.

How to use a handheld resuscitation bag

Place the mask over the patient's face so the apex of the triangle covers the bridge of his nose and the base lies between his lower lip and chin.

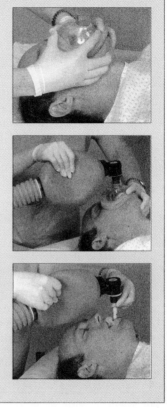

Make sure his mouth remains open underneath the mask. Attach the handheld resuscitation bag to the face mask and the oxygen source.

If the patient has a tracheostomy or endotracheal tube in place, remove the mask from the bag and attach the handheld resuscitation bag directly to the tube using an appropriate adapter, if necessary.

■ Monitor the patient's oxygen saturation level, if available, to make sure that adequate ventilation and oxygen concentration is given.

SPECIAL CONSIDERATIONS
■ Avoid neck hyperextension if the patient has a possible cervical injury; instead, use the jaw-thrust technique to open the airway.

- If you need both hands to keep the mask in place and maintain hyperextension, use the lower part of your arm to compress the bag against your side or ask another staff member for assistance.
- Observe for vomiting through the clear part of the mask.
- If vomiting occurs, stop immediately, lift the mask, wipe and suction vomitus, and resume resuscitation.
- Reinforce to the patient why manual ventilation is necessary and the procedure involved, if appropriate, to lessen anxiety.

COMPLICATIONS

Aspiration of vomitus can result in pneumonia, and gastric distention may result from air forced into the patient's stomach. Underventilation commonly occurs because the handheld resuscitation bag is difficult to keep positioned tightly on the patient's face while ensuring an open airway.

DOCUMENTATION
Emergency documentation

- Note the date and time of the procedure.
- Record manual ventilation efforts.
- Document any complications and nursing action taken.
- Note the patient's response to treatment, according to your facility's protocol for respiratory arrest.
- Document the patient's oxygen saturation level during manual ventilation, and the concentration of oxygen given.

Nonemergency documentation

- Note the date and time of the procedure.
- Record the reason and length of time the patient was disconnected from mechanical ventilation and received manual ventilation.
- Document any complications and nursing action taken.
- Note the patient's tolerance of the procedure.
- Document the patient's oxygen saturation level during the procedure, and the concentration of oxygen given.

Mechanical ventilation

A mechanical ventilator moves air in and out of lungs. Mechanical ventilation is used for acute respiratory failure due to such conditions as acute respiratory distress syndrome, pneumonia, heart failure, or trauma. It may also be used to treat respiratory center depression due to stroke, brain injury, or trauma. The main types of mechanical ventilation systems are positive-pressure, negative-pressure, and high-frequency ventilation.

Positive-pressure systems, the most commonly used, can be volume-cycled or pressure-cycled. Negative-pressure systems (such as the iron lung) provide ventilation for patients who can't generate adequate inspiratory pressures such as patients with neuromuscular disorders. High-frequency ventilation systems provide high ventilation rates with low peak airway pressures, synchronized to the patient's own inspiratory efforts.

EQUIPMENT

Positive-pressure or negative-pressure ventilator ● oxygen saturation monitor ● handheld resuscitation bag with the appropriate adapter

PREPARATION OF EQUIPMENT

■ In most facilities, a respiratory therapist sets up the ventilator.
■ In most cases, the respiratory therapist will also add sterile distilled water to the humidifier and connect the ventilator to the appropriate gas source.
■ Make sure that the ventilator is connected to an uninterruptible or emergency power source.

ESSENTIAL STEPS

■ Review and be familiar with the physician's orders for mechanical ventilation.
■ Connect a handheld resuscitation bag to an oxygen source and place it at the bedside.
■ Put on gloves and personal protective equipment.
■ Place the oxygen saturation monitor, if available, on the patient.
■ Assist the registered nurse, physician, or respiratory therapist to connect the endotracheal tube to the ventilator.
■ Observe the patient for chest expansion and monitor for bilateral breath sounds.
■ Monitor the patient's oxygen saturation level or arterial blood gas (ABG) values 20 to 30 minutes after the initial ventilator setup and any changes in ventilator settings, and as patient's clinical condition warrants, according to the physician's order.
■ The physician will order adjustments in ventilator settings depending on ABG results and, in most facilities, the respiratory therapist will perform the changes.
■ Check the ventilator tubing for condensation.

- Condensation shouldn't be left to collect in the tubing or drained into the humidifier. It should be drained into a collection trap and emptied.
- Monitor the in-line thermometer to make sure the air is close to body temperature.
- When monitoring the patient's vital signs, count spontaneous and ventilator-delivered breaths.
- The respiratory therapist will change, clean, or dispose of the ventilator tubing and equipment every 48 to 72 hours to reduce risk of bacterial contamination.
- When ordered, the patient will begin to be weaned from the ventilator.

SPECIAL CONSIDERATIONS

- Make sure ventilator alarms and oxygen saturation monitor, if available, are on at all times. (See *Responding to ventilator alarms,* pages 116 and 117.)
- If a ventilator alarm sounds and the problem can't be identified, disconnect the patient from the ventilator and use a handheld resuscitation bag to ventilate him. Contact the registered nurse, physician, and respiratory therapist immediately.
- Provide reassurance even if the patient is unresponsive.
- Keep the head of the patient's bed elevated to at least 30 degrees to help prevent hospital-acquired pneumonia.
- Unless contraindicated, turn the patient from side to side every 1 to 2 hours.

RED FLAG When moving a patient or the ventilator tubing, be careful to prevent condensation in the tubing from flowing into the lungs because aspiration of this contaminated moisture can cause infection.

- Perform active or passive range-of-motion exercises.
- If permitted, position the patient upright at regular intervals.
- Provide care for the patient's artificial airway as needed and according to your facility's policy.
- Monitor peripheral circulation and urine output.
- Monitor for fluid volume excess or dehydration.
- Place the call bell within reach.
- Establish a method of communication such as a communication board.
- Monitor the patient for signs of anxiety and spontaneous breathing efforts that interfere with the ventilator's action. A sedative or neuromuscular blocker may need to be given.
- Make sure that emergency equipment is readily available.

■ Reinforce the explanation of all procedures and ensure patient safety.

■ Make sure that the patient gets adequate rest and sleep.

■ Provide subdued lighting, low noise, and restricted staff.

■ Observe for signs of hypoxia when the patient is being weaned.

■ With the patient's input, help schedule weaning around his daily regimen.

■ As weaning progresses, encourage and assist the patient to get out of bed as ordered.

■ Plan diversionary activities to take his mind off breathing.

■ During and after intubation, provide frequent mouth care because the patient's mucous membranes, tongue, and lips may become irritated, dry, and cracked.

■ For home use, reinforce the teaching plan that covers ventilator care and settings, artificial airway care, suctioning, respiratory therapy, communication, nutrition, therapeutic exercise, signs and symptoms of infection, and troubleshooting minor equipment malfunctions.

■ Observe as the caregiver demonstrates the ability to use the equipment.

■ Make sure the patient has a referral to a home health agency, a durable medical equipment vendor, and community resources.

COMPLICATIONS

Mechanical ventilation can cause traumatic tension pneumothorax, decreased cardiac output, oxygen toxicity, fluid volume excess (caused by humidification), infection, and GI complications, such as distention or bleeding from stress ulcers.

DOCUMENTATION

■ Record the date and time of initiation of mechanical ventilation.

■ Note the name, type, and settings of the ventilator.

■ Document the patient's responses to mechanical ventilation, including vital signs, breath sounds, use of accessory muscles, intake and output, and weight.

■ Record any complications and nursing actions taken.

■ Note pertinent laboratory data.

■ Document the weaning date, time, method, vital signs, oxygen saturation levels, and ABG values.

■ Note the patient's level of consciousness, respiratory effort, spontaneous breathing, arrhythmias, skin color, and need for suctioning.

■ Note the amount, color, consistency, and odor of secretions.

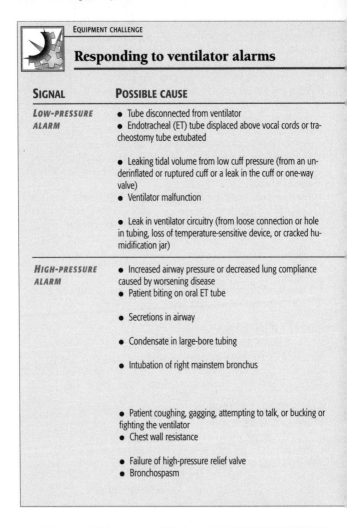

Responding to ventilator alarms

SIGNAL	POSSIBLE CAUSE
LOW-PRESSURE ALARM	• Tube disconnected from ventilator • Endotracheal (ET) tube displaced above vocal cords or tracheostomy tube extubated • Leaking tidal volume from low cuff pressure (from an underinflated or ruptured cuff or a leak in the cuff or one-way valve) • Ventilator malfunction • Leak in ventilator circuitry (from loose connection or hole in tubing, loss of temperature-sensitive device, or cracked humidification jar)
HIGH-PRESSURE ALARM	• Increased airway pressure or decreased lung compliance caused by worsening disease • Patient biting on oral ET tube • Secretions in airway • Condensate in large-bore tubing • Intubation of right mainstem bronchus • Patient coughing, gagging, attempting to talk, or bucking or fighting the ventilator • Chest wall resistance • Failure of high-pressure relief valve • Bronchospasm

Mucus clearance

A mucus clearance device is used for patients who need mucus secretions removed from the lungs and those with chronic respiratory disorders. A handheld mucus clearance device (known as *the flutter*)

NURSING INTERVENTIONS

- Reconnect the tube to the ventilator.
- Check the tube placement and have the physician or respiratory therapist reposition it if needed. If extubation or displacement has occurred, ventilate the patient manually and call the physician immediately.
- Listen for a whooshing, grunting, or crowing sound around tube, indicating an air leak. If you hear one, check cuff pressure. If you can't maintain pressure, call the physician; he may need to insert a new tube.
- Disconnect the patient from the ventilator and ventilate him manually if necessary. Obtain another ventilator.
- Make sure all connections are intact. Check for holes, leaks, or dislodged caps in the tubing and replace the caps or tubing if necessary. Check the humidification jar and replace if cracked.

- Monitor the patient's respiratory status for evidence of increasing lung consolidation, barotrauma, or wheezing. Call the physician if indicated.
- Insert an oral airway if needed.
- The physician may consider an analgesic or sedative, if appropriate.
- Look for secretions in the airway. To remove them, suction the patient or have him cough.
- Check the tubing for condensate and remove any fluid. Don't drain the condensate back into the humidifier.
- Monitor the patient's respiratory status for evidence of diminished or absent breath sounds in the left lung fields.
- Check the tube position. If it has slipped, call the physician; he may need to reposition it.
- If the patient fights the ventilator, the physician may order a sedative or neuromuscular blocker.
- Reposition the patient to improve chest expansion. If repositioning doesn't help, give the prescribed analgesic. To give an I.V. analgesic, call the registered nurse.
- Have faulty equipment replaced.
- Report to the physician and treat as ordered.

helps patients cough up secretions more easily. (See *Flutter valve device*, page 118.) Vibrations propagate throughout airway during expiration, loosening the mucus. Mucus progressively moves up the airways until it can be coughed out easily.

Flutter valve device

When the patient exhales through the flutter valve device, both positive end-expiratory pressure and high-frequency oscillations help move mucus.

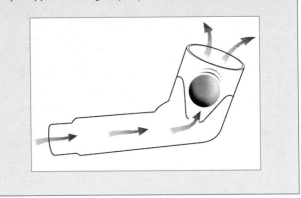

CONTRAINDICATIONS
■ Don't use this device in a patient with an ineffective cough reflex.

EQUIPMENT
Mucus clearance device ● emesis basin ● tissues ● pulse oximeter

ESSENTIAL STEPS
■ Reinforce the explanation of the steps of the procedure to the patient.
■ Remind the patient that this device will move mucus through his airway so he can eventually expectorate it.
■ Position the patient sitting with his back straight and his head tilted back slightly to open his throat and trachea.
■ If the patient places his elbows on a table, the height should prevent slouching.
■ Have the patient hold the device so that the stem is horizontal, draw a deep breath, hold it for 2 to 3 seconds, place the device in his mouth and exhale at a steady rate for as long as possible.
■ Quick or forceful exhalations prevent vibration and flutter.
■ Remind the patient to keep his cheeks as flat and hard as possible while exhaling.

- To reinforce teaching related to the technique, have the patient hold his cheeks lightly with his other hand.
- After the patient exhales completely, he should remove the device from his mouth, take in another full breath, and cough. Repeat several times.
- Alternatively, after completely exhaling, the patient can leave the device in his mouth, draw another full breath through his nose, hold it for 2 to 3 seconds, and repeat the exhalation maneuver.
- The patient can breathe through the device up to five times before taking the final breath and coughing.
- Provide an emesis basin and tissues.

SPECIAL CONSIDERATIONS

- To help the patient achieve the best fluttering effect, place one hand on his back and the other on his chest as he exhales through the device.
- If the patient is achieving the maximum effect, you'll feel vibrations in his lungs as he exhales.
- If results are unsatisfactory at first, tell the patient to adjust the angle at which he's holding the device until optimal fluttering occurs.
- If the patient's final cough doesn't seem to work, he can try repeated, controlled, short, rapid exhalations to aid mucus removal.
- After the procedure, thoroughly clean the device. All parts should be rinsed under a stream of hot tap water, wiped with a clean towel, reassembled, and stored in a clean, dry place.
- Monitor the patient's respiratory status.
- Reinforce why the procedure is necessary, how to use the device, how to clean the device after each use (reminding the patient to clean it more thoroughly every 2 days in a solution of mild soap or detergent), and how to use controlled, short, rapid exhalations to help remove loosened mucus.
- Encourage adequate hydration to liquefy and thin secretions.
- Reinforce that the patient should avoid milk and milk products, which tend to make secretions more difficult to remove.

COMPLICATIONS

This technique may cause a mucus plug to become lodged in the patient's airway.

DOCUMENTATION
▪ Document the amount, color, consistency, and odor of secretions, the patient's respiratory status before and after the procedure, and how he tolerated the procedure.
▪ Record the number of repetitions and success level of coughing efforts.
▪ Note the patient's ability to demonstrate use of the device.
▪ Document the patient's oxygen saturation level before and after the procedure.

Nebulizer therapy

Nebulizer therapy aids bronchial hygiene by restoring and maintaining mucous blanket continuity, hydrating dried secretions, promoting secretion expectoration, humidifying inspired oxygen, and delivering drugs. It may be given through nebulizers that have large or small volume, are ultrasonic, or are placed inside ventilator tubing. Large-volume nebulizers (such as a Venturi jet) provide humidity for an artificial airway. Small-volume nebulizers (such as a mininebulizer) are used to deliver drugs such as bronchodilators. Ultrasonic nebulizers are electrically driven and use high-frequency vibrations to break up surface water into particles; resultant dense mist can penetrate smaller airways, hydrate secretions, and induce coughing. In-line nebulizers are used to deliver drugs to patients being mechanically ventilated.

CONTRAINDICATIONS
None known.

EQUIPMENT
For an ultrasonic nebulizer
Ultrasonic gas-delivery device ● large-bore oxygen tubing ● nebulizer couplet compartment

For a large-volume nebulizer
Pressurized gas source ● flowmeter ● large-bore oxygen tubing ● nebulizer bottle ● sterile distilled water ● heater (if ordered) ● in-line thermometer (if using heater)

For a small-volume nebulizer
Pressurized gas source ● flowmeter ● oxygen tubing ● nebulizer cup ● mouthpiece or mask ● normal saline solution ● prescribed drug

For an in-line nebulizer
Pressurized gas source ● flowmeter ● nebulizer cup ● normal saline solution ● prescribed drug

PREPARATION OF EQUIPMENT
For an ultrasonic nebulizer
■ Fill the couplet compartment to the indicated level.

For a large-volume nebulizer
■ Fill with distilled water to the indicated level.
■ Avoid using normal saline solution, to prevent corrosion.
■ Add a heating device if ordered.
■ Ensure delivery of the prescribed oxygen percentage.

For a small-volume nebulizer
■ Draw up the drug, inject it into the nebulizer cup, and add the prescribed amount of normal saline solution, or water.
■ Attach the mouthpiece, mask, or other gas-delivery device.

For an in-line nebulizer
■ Draw up the drug and diluent, remove the nebulizer cup, quickly inject the drug, then replace the cup.
■ If using an intermittent positive-pressure breathing machine, attach the mouthpiece and mask to the machine.

ESSENTIAL STEPS
■ Identify the patient using two patient identifiers, such as the patient's name and identification number.
■ Reinforce the explanation of the procedure to the patient.
■ Wash your hands.
■ Take the patient's vital signs and monitor his respiratory status.
■ Place the patient in a sitting or high Fowler's position.

For an ultrasonic nebulizer
■ Give an inhaled bronchodilator to prevent bronchospasm.
■ Turn the machine on and check the outflow port for proper misting.
■ Monitor the patient for adverse reactions.
■ Watch for labored respirations.
■ Take the patient's vital signs and monitor his respiratory status.
■ Encourage the patient to cough and expectorate, or suction him as needed.

For a large-volume nebulizer
■ Attach the delivery device to the patient.
■ Encourage the patient to cough and expectorate, or suction him as needed.
■ Check the water level in the nebulizer and refill it, as indicated.
■ When refilling a reusable container, discard the old water.
■ Change the nebulizer unit and tubing according to your facility's policy.
■ If the nebulizer is heated, tell the patient to report discomfort.
■ Use the in-line thermometer to monitor the temperature of the gas the patient is inhaling.
■ If you turn off the flow for more than 5 minutes, unplug the heater.

For a small-volume nebulizer
■ Attach the flowmeter to the gas source.
■ Attach the nebulizer to the flowmeter and adjust the flow to at least 10 L.
■ Check the outflow port to ensure adequate misting.
■ Remain with the patient during treatment.
■ Take the patient's vital signs and monitor him for adverse reactions.
■ Encourage the patient to cough and expectorate, or suction him as necessary.
■ Change the nebulizer cup and tubing according to your facility's policy.

For an in-line nebulizer
■ Turn on the machine and check for proper misting.
■ Remain with the patient during treatment.
■ Take the patient's vital signs and monitor him for adverse reactions.
■ Encourage the patient to cough, and suction excess secretions as necessary.
■ Monitor the patient's respiratory status to evaluate the effectiveness of therapy.

SPECIAL CONSIDERATIONS
■ The efficacy of aerosol therapy, what type of fluids to use, the types of drugs that can be delivered, and the effectiveness of therapy, haven't been established.
■ Monitor for overhydration, especially in the patient with a delicate fluid balance.

LIFE STAGES *Pediatric patients are especially at risk for over-hydration from nebulizer therapy. It may provide a relatively large increase in fluid volume in these patients.*

■ Carefully monitor for adequate flow if oxygen is being delivered at the same time.
■ Encourage the patient to take slow, even breaths to derive maximum benefit.

COMPLICATIONS
Nebulizer therapy can cause mucosa irritation, bronchospasm, dyspnea, airway burns, infection, and adverse drug reactions.

DOCUMENTATION
■ Record the date, time, and duration of therapy.
■ Note the type and amount of drug given.
■ Document the fraction of inspired oxygen or oxygen flow.
■ Record baseline and subsequent vital signs and a description of the patient's baseline and postprocedure respiratory status.
■ Note the patient's response to treatment.
■ Record any adverse reactions, the treatments ordered and given, and the patient's response.

Pulse oximetry

Pulse oximetry is used to noninvasively monitor arterial oxygen saturation. A photodetector slipped over the finger measures transmitted light as it passes through the vascular bed, detects the relative amount of color absorbed by arterial blood, and calculates exact mixed venous oxygen saturation without interference from surrounding venous blood, skin, connective tissue, or bone. (See *How oximetry works,* page 124.)

CONTRAINDICATIONS
None known.

EQUIPMENT
Oximeter ● sensor probe ● alcohol pads ● nail polish remover, if necessary

PREPARATION OF EQUIPMENT
■ Review the manufacturer's instructions for assembly.

How oximetry works

The pulse oximeter allows noninvasive monitoring of a patient's arterial oxygen saturation levels by measuring absorption (amplitude) of light waves as they pass through areas of the body that are highly perfused by arterial blood. Oximetry also monitors pulse rate and amplitude.

Light-emitting diodes in a transducer (photodetector) attached to the patient's body (shown at right on index finger) send red and infrared light beams through tissue. The photodetector records the relative amount of each color absorbed by arterial blood and transmits the data to a monitor, which displays the information with each heartbeat. If the oxygen saturation level or pulse rate varies from preset limits, the monitor triggers visual and audible alarms.

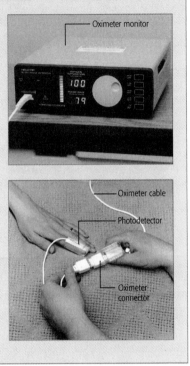

Oximeter monitor

Oximeter cable

Photodetector

Oximeter connector

ESSENTIAL STEPS

■ Reinforce the explanation of the procedure to the patient.

Using a finger probe

■ Select a finger (usually index finger) on the patient's nondominant hand, if possible for placement of the probe.
■ Remove fake fingernail and nail polish from the test finger.
■ Place the transducer (photodetector) probe over the patient's finger so the light beams and sensors oppose each other.
■ Trim long fingernails or position the probe perpendicular to the finger.
■ Position the patient's hand at heart level.

LIFE STAGES *If testing a neonate or small infant, wrap the probe around the foot so the light beams and detectors oppose each other. For a large infant, use a probe that fits on the great toe and secure it to the foot.*

■ Turn on the power switch. If the device is working properly, a beep will sound, a display will light momentarily, and the pulse searchlight will flash.

■ After four to six heartbeats the pulse amplitude indicator will begin tracking the pulse.

■ Rotate the sensor site according to the manufacturer's instructions and your facility's policy to prevent skin irritation and circulatory impairment.

■ Clean the probe per facility policy between patients or, if disposable, discard.

SPECIAL CONSIDERATIONS

■ Some machines have a pleth wave. A steady, level, even waveform ensures that the numerical reading is accurate.

■ The pulse rate on the oximeter should correspond to the patient's actual pulse. If it doesn't, monitor the patient, check the oximeter, and reposition the probe.

■ Factors that interfere with accuracy include:
  – elevated carboxyhemoglobin or methemoglobin levels
  – lipid emulsions and dyes
  – excessive light
  – excessive patient movement
  – hypothermia
  – hypotension
  – vasoconstriction
  – medications (such as dapsone, vasopressors).

■ Use the bridge of the nose if the patient has compromised circulation in his extremities.

■ If an automatic blood pressure cuff is used on the same extremity as the saturation probe is placed, the cuff will interfere with oxygen saturation readings during inflation.

■ If light is a problem, cover the probes.

■ If patient movement is a problem, move the probe or select a different probe. (See *Identifying pulse oximeter problems,* page 126.)

■ Normal SpO_2 levels for pulse oximetry are 95% to 100% for adults and 93.8% to 100% by 1 hour after birth for healthy, full-term neonates.

■ Lower levels may indicate hypoxemia that warrants intervention.

EQUIPMENT CHALLENGE

Identifying pulse oximeter problems

To maintain a continuous display of arterial oxygen saturation levels, keep the monitoring site clean and dry. Make sure the skin doesn't become irritated from adhesives used to keep disposable probes in place. Change the site if this happens. Disposable probes that irritate skin can also be replaced with nondisposable models.

Another common problem with pulse oximeters is failure of the device to obtain a signal. If this happens, first check the patient's vital signs. If they're sufficient to produce a signal, check for the following problems.

POOR CONNECTION
Check that the sensors are properly aligned. Make sure the wires are intact and securely fastened and the pulse oximeter is plugged into a power source.

INADEQUATE OR INTERMITTENT BLOOD FLOW TO SITE
Check the patient's pulse rate and capillary refill time. Take immediate corrective action and notify the physician if blood flow to the site is suddenly decreased. Loosen any restraints, remove tight-fitting clothes, take off a blood pressure cuff, and check arterial and I.V. lines. If none of these interventions work, you may need to find an alternate site. Finding a site with proper circulation may also prove challenging when a patient is receiving vasoconstrictive drugs.

EQUIPMENT MALFUNCTIONS
Remove the pulse oximeter from the patient, set the alarm limits according to your facility's policies, and try the instrument on yourself or another healthy person. This will tell you if the equipment is working correctly.

■ Notify the physician of any significant change in the patient's condition.

COMPLICATIONS
None known.

DOCUMENTATION
■ Note the procedure, date, time, oxygen saturation level, and actions taken.
■ Record the oxygen saturation reading on appropriate flowcharts, if indicated.
■ Record oxygen therapy in use at the time of the reading.

Thoracentesis assistance

A thoracentesis relieves pulmonary compression and respiratory distress by removing air or fluid, which has accumulated as a result of injury or a condition such as tuberculosis or cancer, from the pleural space. Thoracentesis provides a specimen of pleural fluid or tissue for analysis and allows for the instillation of chemotherapeutic agents or other drugs into the pleural space.

CONTRAINDICATIONS
■ A known bleeding disorder.

EQUIPMENT
Most facilities use a prepackaged thoracentesis tray.

Sterile gloves ● sterile drapes ● 70% isopropyl alcohol or povidone-iodine solution ● 1% or 2% lidocaine ● 5-ml syringe with 21G and 25G needles for anesthetic injection ● 17G thoracentesis needle for aspiration ● 50-ml syringe ● three-way stopcock and tubing ● sterile specimen containers ● sterile hemostat ● sterile 4″ × 4″ gauze pads ● adhesive tape ● sphygmomanometer ● gloves ● stethoscope ● laboratory request forms ● drainage bottles ● shaving supplies ● biopsy needle ● prescribed sedative with 3-ml syringe and 21G needle ● drainage bottles (if the physician expects a large amount of drainage) ● Teflon catheter (optional)

PREPARATION OF EQUIPMENT
■ Assemble all equipment at the patient's bedside or treatment area.
■ Check the expiration date on each sterile package and inspect for tears.
■ Prepare the laboratory request form, listing current antibiotics (this will be considered when the specimens are analyzed).
■ Make sure the patient has a signed consent form. Note drug allergies, especially to the local anesthetic and latex.
■ Place recent chest X-rays at the bedside.

ESSENTIAL STEPS
■ Identify the patient using two patient identifiers, such as the patient's name and identification number.
■ Reinforce the explanation of the procedure to the patient. Remind him that he may feel discomfort and a sensation of pressure during needle insertion.
■ Provide privacy and emotional support.
■ Wash your hands.

■ Determine whether the patient needs a sedative or analgesic before the procedure.

■ Obtain the patient's baseline vital signs and oxygen saturation level, and monitor his respiratory status.

■ Position the patient on the edge of the bed with his legs supported and his head and folded arms resting on a pillow on the overbed table; alternatively, have him straddle a chair backward and rest his head and folded arms on the back of the chair.

■ If the patient can't sit, turn him on the unaffected side with the arm of the affected side raised above his head.

■ Elevate the head of the bed 30 to 45 degrees if not contraindicated. Proper positioning stretches the chest or back and allows easier access to intercostal spaces.

■ The team should take a "time out" to verify that the right procedure is being performed on the right patient at the right site.

■ Remind the patient not to cough, breathe deeply, or move suddenly during the procedure to avoid puncture of the visceral pleura or lung.

RED FLAG *If the patient coughs, the physician will briefly stop the procedure and withdraw the needle slightly to prevent puncture.*

■ Expose the patient's entire chest or back and shave the aspiration site, as ordered.

■ Wash your hands again before touching the sterile equipment.

■ Using sterile technique, open the thoracentesis tray and assist the physician as necessary to disinfect the site.

■ If an ampule of local anesthetic isn't included in the sterile tray and a multidose vial of local anesthetic will be used, assist the physician by wiping the rubber stopper with an alcohol pad and holding the inverted vial while the physician inserts the needle into the stopper and withdraws the anesthetic solution.

■ After draping the patient and injecting the local anesthetic, the physician will attach a three-way stopcock with tubing to the aspirating needle and turn the stopcock to prevent air from entering the pleural space through the needle.

■ Attach the other end of the tubing to the drainage bottle.

■ The physician will insert the needle into the pleural space and attach a 50-ml syringe to the needle's stopcock.

■ A hemostat may be used to hold the needle in place and help prevent a pleural tear or lung puncture. Alternatively, the physician may introduce a Teflon catheter into the needle, remove the needle, and attach a stopcock and syringe or drainage tubing to the catheter to reduce the risk of pleural puncture by the needle.

■ Check the patient's vital signs regularly during the procedure.

RED FLAG Watch for signs of distress, such as pallor, vertigo, faintness, weak and rapid pulse, decreased blood pressure, dyspnea, tachypnea, diaphoresis, chest pain, blood-tinged mucus, and excessive coughing. Alert the physician because these signs may indicate hypovolemic shock, tension pneumothorax, or other complication.

■ Put on gloves and assist the physician as necessary to collect necessary specimens, drain fluid, and dress the site.

■ After the physician withdraws the needle or catheter, apply pressure to the puncture site using a sterile 4″ × 4″ gauze pad.

■ Apply a new sterile gauze pad and secure it with tape.

■ Place the patient in a comfortable position, take his vital signs, and monitor his oxygen saturation level and respiratory status.

■ Label the specimens properly and send them to the laboratory.

■ Discard disposable equipment. Clean nondisposable items and return them for sterilization.

■ Check vital signs, oxygen saturation level, and the dressing for drainage every 15 minutes for 1 hour; continue to monitor as indicated by the patient's condition.

■ Have the patient maintain bed rest after the procedure if prescribed.

SPECIAL CONSIDERATIONS

■ Monitor the amount of drainage closely.

RED FLAG To prevent pulmonary edema and hypovolemic shock after thoracentesis, the physician will remove fluid slowly (no more than 1,000 ml of fluid during the first 30 minutes). Removing fluid increases negative intrapleural pressure, which can lead to edema if the lung doesn't reexpand to fill the space.

■ Pleuritic or shoulder pain may indicate pleural irritation by the needle point.

■ A chest X-ray is usually ordered after the procedure to detect pneumothorax and evaluate the results of the procedure.

■ The patient may experience some coughing after the procedure.

■ Reinforce the explanation of the procedure to the patient, keep him informed of each step, watch for signs of anxiety, and provide reassurance as necessary.

COMPLICATIONS

Complications of a thoracentesis include pneumothorax (possibly leading to mediastinal shift and requiring chest tube insertion) if the needle punctures the lung and allows air to enter the pleural cavity, pyogenic infection from contamination, pain, anxiety, dry taps, and subcutaneous hematoma.

DOCUMENTATION

■ Record the date and time of thoracentesis and the name of the physician who performed the procedure.

■ Note the location and a description of the puncture site.

■ Document the volume and description (color, viscosity, odor) of fluid withdrawn.

■ Record specimens sent to the laboratory.

■ Note the patient's vital signs and oxygen saturation level, and describe his respiratory status before, during, and after the procedure.

■ Document postprocedural tests, such as chest X-rays, and any medications given.

■ Record any complications and nursing actions taken.

■ Note the patient's response to the procedure.

Thoracic drainage

Thoracic drainage uses gravity, and possibly suction, to remove accumulated air, fluids (blood, pus, chyle, and serous fluids), or solids (blood clots) from the pleural cavity and restore negative pressure, which reexpands a partially or totally collapsed lung. A disposable drainage system combines drainage collection, a water seal, and suction control into a single unit. The underwater seal in the drainage system allows air and fluid to escape from the pleural cavity but doesn't allow air to reenter.

CONTRAINDICATIONS

None known.

EQUIPMENT

Thoracic drainage system (for example, Pleur-evac, Argyle [which can function as a gravity draining system or be connected to suction to enhance chest drainage]) ● sterile distilled water ● elastic tape ● sterile clear plastic tubing ● bottle or system rack ● two rubber-tipped Kelly clamps ● sterile 50-ml catheter-tip syringe ● suction source, if ordered ● rubber band or safety pin

PREPARATION OF EQUIPMENT

■ Check the physician's order to determine the type of drainage system to be used and specific procedural details.

■ Take the appropriate equipment to the patient's bedside.

■ Wash your hands.

■ Maintain sterile technique throughout the procedure.

- Open the packaged system and place it on the floor in the rack supplied by the manufacturer to avoid accidentally knocking it over or dislodging the components.
- Remove the plastic connector from the short tube attached to the water-seal chamber.
- Using a 50-ml catheter-tip syringe, instill sterile distilled water into the water-seal chamber until it reaches the 2-cm mark or the mark specified by the manufacturer, facility, or physician.
- Replace the plastic connector.
- If suction is ordered, remove the cap (also called the *muffler* or *atmosphere vent cover*) on the suction-control chamber to open the vent.
- Instill sterile distilled water until it reaches the 20-cm mark or the ordered level and recap the suction-control chamber.
- After the system is prepared, hang it from the bed frame (not the side rail).

ESSENTIAL STEPS

- Reinforce the explanation of the procedure to the patient and wash your hands.
- Maintaining sterile technique, use the long tube to connect the patient's chest tube to the closed drainage collection chamber and secure the connection with tape.
- Connect the short tube on the drainage system to the suction source and turn on the suction.
- Gentle bubbling should begin in the suction chamber, indicating that the correct suction level has been reached.
- Note the character, consistency, and amount of drainage in the drainage collection chamber.
- Mark the drainage level in the drainage collection chamber with the time and date every 8 hours (or more often if there's a large amount of drainage), according to your facility's policy, or according to physician's order.
- Check the water level in the water-seal chamber every 8 hours. If necessary, carefully add sterile distilled water until the level reaches the 2-cm mark indicated on the water-seal chamber of the commercial system.
- Check for fluctuation in the water-seal chamber as the patient breathes.
- Normal fluctuations of 2″ to 4″ (5 to 10 cm) reflect pressure changes in the pleural space during respiration.
- To check for fluctuation with a suction system, momentarily disconnect the suction system so the air vent is opened and observe for fluctuation.

- Check for intermittent bubbling in the water-seal chamber. This usually occurs when the system is removing air from the pleural cavity. If bubbling isn't readily apparent during quiet breathing, have the patient take a deep breath or cough. Absence of bubbling indicates that the pleural space has sealed.
- Check for gentle bubbling in the suction control chamber; this indicates that the proper suction level has been reached. Vigorous bubbling in this chamber increases the rate of water evaporation. Periodically check that the air vent in the system is working properly.

RED FLAG *Occlusion of the air vent results in a buildup of pressure in the system that could cause the patient to develop tension pneumothorax.*

- Check the water level in the suction-control chamber. Detach the chamber from the suction source; when bubbling ceases, observe the water level. If needed, add sterile distilled water to bring the level to the 20-cm line or as ordered. If water needs to be removed, use sterile technique and a needle and syringe to draw it out of the injection port located at the bottom of the suction chamber.
- Keep the drainage tubing at the level of the patient. Avoid creating dependent loops, kinks, or pressure on the tubing. Avoid lifting the drainage system above the patient's chest because fluid may flow back into the pleural space.
- Keep two rubber-tipped clamps at the bedside to clamp the chest tube as close to the patient as possible if the commercially prepared system cracks or to locate an air leak in the system.
- Encourage the patient to use an incentive spirometer and to cough frequently and breathe deeply.
- Remind the patient to sit upright and splint the insertion site while coughing to minimize pain.
- Check the patient's respiratory status periodically to monitor air exchange in the affected lung. Diminished or absent breath sounds may indicate that the lung hasn't reexpanded.

RED FLAG *Reinforce that the patient should report difficulty breathing immediately. Notify the physician immediately if the patient develops cyanosis, rapid or shallow breathing, subcutaneous emphysema, chest pain, or excessive bleeding.*

- When clots are visible you may be able to milk the tubing, depending on your facility's policy. Gently milk tubing in the direction of the drainage chamber as needed.
- Check the chest tube dressing at least every 8 hours and change it if necessary, according to the physician's orders and your facility's policy.

▶ *RED FLAG Palpate the area surrounding the dressing for crepitus or subcutaneous emphysema, which indicates that air is leaking into the subcutaneous tissue surrounding the insertion site.*

■ Encourage active or passive range-of-motion (ROM) exercises for the patient's arm or the affected side if he has been splinting the insertion site.

■ Reinforce that the patient should ask for analgesics as needed for comfort and to help with deep breathing, coughing, and ROM exercises. Monitor for signs and symptoms of discomfort such as grimacing.

■ Remind the ambulatory patient to keep the drainage system below chest level and to be careful not to disconnect the tubing to maintain the water seal. Encourage him to ask for assistance when getting out of bed.

SPECIAL CONSIDERATIONS

■ Before transferring the patient or allowing him to ambulate, review the physician's orders. He may order that the patient not be removed from suction at any time.

■ If excessive continuous bubbling is present in the water-seal chamber, especially if suction is being used, rule out a leak in the drainage system.

Assisting with locating an air leak

■ To locate a leak, the tube is momentarily clamped at various points along its length.

■ Clamping begins at the proximal end of the tube, working down toward the drainage system, with special attention to the seal around the connections.

■ If a connection is loose, push it back together and tape it securely.

■ Bubbling will stop when a clamp is placed between the air leak and the water seal. If the tube is clamped along the entire length and bubbling doesn't stop, the drainage unit may be cracked and need replacement.

■ If the drainage collection chamber fills or the system cracks, it will need to be replaced. Follow your facility's policy for replacing the collection chamber. In most cases, to replace the chamber, the chest tube is double-clamped close to the insertion site (using two clamps facing in opposite directions), the system is exchanged, the clamps are removed, and the connection is re-taped.

RED FLAG *Never leave the chest tube clamped for more than 1 minute to prevent tension pneumothorax, which may occur when air and fluid are kept from escaping.*

■ Observe the patient for altered respirations while the tube is clamped.

■ Instead of clamping the tube, you may submerge the distal end of the tube in a container of sterile normal saline solution placed at a level lower than the patient's lung to create a temporary water seal while you replace the drainage system. Check your facility's policy for the proper procedure.

■ Encourage the patient to report difficulty breathing immediately.

COMPLICATIONS

Tension pneumothorax can occur as a result of thoracic drainage.

DOCUMENTATION

■ Note the date and time thoracic drainage was initiated and the type of system used.

■ Record the amount of suction applied to the pleural cavity.

■ Note the presence or absence of bubbling or fluctuation in the water-seal chamber.

■ Record the initial amount and type of drainage, and document a description of the patient's respiratory status.

■ Note the frequency of system inspection and record how often chest tubes were milked (if congruent with your facility's policy).

■ Document amount, color, and consistency of drainage; note the condition of the chest dressings.

■ Document if analgesics were given.

■ Document any complications and nursing actions taken.

■ Document the date and time that chest X-rays are taken.

■ Record oxygen therapy in use and oxygen saturation levels, if available.

Tracheal suction

In the tracheal suction procedure, secretions from the trachea or bronchi are removed by means of a catheter inserted through the mouth or nose, tracheal stoma, a tracheostomy tube, or an endotracheal (ET) tube. Suctioning stimulates the cough reflex and helps maintain a patent airway; it's done as frequently as the patient's condition warrants and as per the physician's order and calls for strict sterile technique.

CONTRAINDICATIONS

■ Check the physician's orders; there may be specific orders regarding tracheal suctioning for patients with severely increased intracranial pressure (ICP).

EQUIPMENT

Oxygen source (wall or portable unit) ● handheld resuscitation bag with a mask or ET or tracheostomy tube with the appropriate adapter, or a positive end-expiratory pressure (PEEP) valve, if indicated ● wall or portable suction apparatus ● collection container ● connecting tube ● suction catheter kit or a sterile suction catheter, one sterile glove, one clean glove, goggles, and a disposable sterile solution container ● 1-L bottle of sterile water or normal saline solution ● sterile water-soluble lubricant (for nasal insertion) ● syringe for deflating cuff of ET or tracheostomy tube ● waterproof trash bag ● sterile towel (optional)

PREPARATION OF EQUIPMENT

■ Choose the appropriate size suction catheter; the diameter should be no larger than one-half the inside diameter of the tracheostomy or ET tube to minimize hypoxia during suctioning. (A #12 or #14 French catheter may be used for an 8-mm or larger tube.)
■ Place the suction apparatus on the patient's overbed table or bedside stand.
■ Attach the collection container to the suction unit with one end of the connecting tube to the collection container; use the end at the patient's bedside for suctioning.
■ Set the suction pressure according to your facility's policy (typically between 80 and 120 mm Hg).
■ Occlude the suction port to assess suction pressure.
■ Label and date the normal saline solution or sterile water and collection container. These should be replaced every 24 hours or according to your facility's policy.
■ Open the waterproof trash bag.
■ If the handheld resuscitation bag will be used for preoxygenation, make sure that it's attached to the oxygen source, set the flow rate at 15 L/minute, and attach the PEEP valve, if necessary.

ESSENTIAL STEPS

■ Obtain a physician's order if required.
■ Monitor the patient's vital signs, oxygen saturation level, respiratory status, and level of consciousness to establish a baseline.

■ Review arterial blood gas values if available.

■ Evaluate the patient's ability to cough and deep breathe.

■ If performing nasotracheal suctioning, check for a deviated septum, nasal polyps, nasal obstruction, nasal trauma, epistaxis, or mucosal swelling.

■ Wash your hands and put on protective equipment.

■ Unless contraindicated, place the patient in semi-Fowler's or high Fowler's position.

■ Remove the top from the normal saline solution or water bottle, open the package containing the sterile solution container, and open the water-soluble lubricant package.

■ Using strict sterile technique, open the suction catheter kit and put on gloves.

■ If using individual supplies, open the suction catheter and the gloves, placing the nonsterile glove on your nondominant hand, then the sterile glove on your dominant hand.

■ Using your nondominant (nonsterile) hand, pour the normal saline solution or sterile water into the solution container.

■ Place a small amount of water-soluble lubricant on the sterile area to facilitate passage of the catheter during nasotracheal suctioning.

■ Place a sterile towel over the patient's chest to provide an additional sterile area.

■ Using your dominant (sterile) hand, remove the catheter from its wrapper. Keep it coiled so it doesn't touch a nonsterile object.

■ Using your nondominant hand, manipulate the connecting tubing and attach the catheter to the tubing.

■ Dip the catheter tip in normal saline solution to lubricate the outside of the catheter.

■ With the catheter tip in the sterile solution, occlude the control valve with the thumb of your nondominant hand. Suction a small amount of solution through the catheter to lubricate the inside and ease passage of secretions.

■ For nasal insertion, lubricate the tip of the catheter with the sterile, water-soluble lubricant.

■ If the patient isn't intubated or is intubated but not receiving oxygen, instruct him to take three to six deep breaths to minimize or prevent hypoxia during suctioning.

■ If the patient isn't intubated but is receiving oxygen, evaluate his need for preoxygenation. If indicated, tell him to take three to six deep breaths while using his supplemental oxygen.

■ The patient may leave his nasal cannula in one nostril or keep the oxygen mask over his mouth.

- If the patient is being mechanically ventilated, preoxygenate him using either a handheld resuscitation bag, the sigh mode on the ventilator, or by activating the 100% fraction of inspired oxygen (FIO_2) button designed for suctioning in some ventilators.
- To preoxygenate the patient with the handheld resuscitation bag, disconnect the patient from the ventilator and deliver four to six breaths with the resuscitation bag.
- If the patient is breathing spontaneously, deliver the breaths while he inhales.
- If the patient is being maintained on PEEP, use a resuscitation bag with a PEEP valve.
- If it is necessary to preoxygenate using the ventilator, first adjust FIO_2 according to your facility's policy and patient requirements. Then use either the sigh mode or manually deliver four to six breaths.

RED FLAG Be sure to adjust the FIO_2 back to the setting ordered by the physician after suctioning if the ventilator isn't designed to do it automatically.

Nasotracheal insertion in a nonintubated patient

- Disconnect the oxygen from the patient, if applicable.
- Using your nondominant hand, raise the tip of the patient's nose.
- Insert the catheter into his nostril while rolling it between your fingers without applying suction.

RED FLAG To avoid oxygen loss and tissue trauma, don't apply suction during insertion.

- As the patient inhales, quickly advance the catheter as far as possible.
- If the patient coughs as the catheter passes through the larynx, briefly hold the catheter still, then resume advancement when he inhales.
- Observe for gagging or the presence of the coiled catheter in the patient's mouth. If this happens, remove the catheter and let him rest.

Insertion in an intubated patient

- If you're using a closed system, the closed tracheal suctioning technique may be used.
- Using your nonsterile hand, disconnect the patient from the ventilator and then stabilize the tip of the ET tube.

- Using your sterile hand, insert the suction catheter into the artificial airway.
- Advance the catheter without applying suction until you meet resistance.
- If the patient coughs, pause; then resume advancement.

Suctioning the patient

- After inserting the catheter, apply suction intermittently by removing and replacing the thumb of your nondominant hand over the control valve.
- Simultaneously use your dominant hand to withdraw the catheter as you roll it between your thumb and forefinger to prevent tissue damage.

 RED FLAG *To prevent hypoxia, never suction for longer than 10 seconds at a time.*

- If applicable, resume oxygen delivery to hyperoxygenate the patient's lungs before continuing, to prevent or relieve hypoxia.
- Allow the patient to rest for a few minutes and encourage him to cough before the next attempt.
- If secretions are thick, clear the catheter periodically by dipping the tip in the normal saline solution and applying suction.
- Watch for variations in sputum color.
- When sputum contains blood, note whether it's streaked or well mixed.
- If arrhythmias occur, stop suctioning and ventilate the patient.

After suctioning

- Hyperoxygenate the patient maintained on a ventilator with the handheld resuscitation bag or by using the ventilator's sigh mode.
- After suctioning the lower airway, determine the need for upper airway suctioning. If necessary, suction the nose and nasopharynx next, and then the mouth.
- If the cuff of the ET or tracheostomy tube is inflated, suction the upper airway before deflating the cuff with a syringe.

RED FLAG *Always change the catheter and sterile glove before resuctioning the lower airway to avoid introducing microorganisms from the upper airway into the lower airway.*

- Discard the gloves and the catheter in the waterproof trash bag.
- Clear connecting tubing by aspirating the remaining normal saline solution or water.
- Wash your hands.

■ Monitor the patient's respiratory status and oxygen saturation level. Take vital signs, if indicated, to determine the effectiveness of the procedure.

SPECIAL CONSIDERATIONS

■ Raising the patient's nose into the sniffing position helps align the larynx and pharynx.

■ If the patient's condition permits, have an assistant extend his head and neck above his shoulders. His lower jaw may need to be moved up and forward. If he's responsive, ask him to stick out his tongue so he won't swallow the catheter during insertion.

■ During suctioning, the catheter is typically advanced as far as the mainstem bronchi.

■ Using an angled catheter may help you guide the catheter into the left mainstem bronchus.

■ Reinforce the explanation of the procedure and reassure the patient, even if he's unresponsive, to minimize anxiety, promote relaxation, and decrease oxygen demand.

■ Remind the patient that suctioning usually causes transient coughing or gagging, but that coughing will help remove secretions.

■ With nasotracheal or orotracheal suctioning, remind the patient to attempt to inhale and exhale steadily and to refrain from swallowing; swallowing may cause the catheter to advance into the esophagus instead of the trachea.

COMPLICATIONS

Tracheal suctioning can cause hypoxemia and dyspnea. Anxiety may alter respiratory patterns. Cardiac arrhythmias can occur from hypoxia. Catheter insertion can cause tracheal or bronchial trauma. Hypoxemia, arrhythmias, hypertension, or hypotension can occur in patients with compromised cardiovascular or pulmonary status. Suctioning can cause increased ICP in patients who already have increased ICP. It can also cause laryngospasm or bronchospasm.

DOCUMENTATION

■ Record the date, time, technique, and reason for the procedure.

■ Document the amount, color, and consistency of secretions.

■ Record any complications and nursing actions taken.

■ Record the preoxygenation method and concentration of oxygen used, if any.

Tracheostomy care

Tracheostomy care is required to ensure airway patency by keeping the tube free from mucus buildup, to maintain mucous membrane and skin integrity, to prevent infection, and to provide psychological support. It should be performed using sterile technique until the stoma has healed. For recent tracheotomies, use sterile gloves for all manipulations at the site. After the stoma has healed, clean gloves may be used.

The patient may have one of three types of tracheostomy tube (uncuffed, cuffed, fenestrated), depending on the patient's condition and physician's preference. An uncuffed plastic or metal tube allows air to flow freely around the tracheostomy tube and through the larynx, reducing the risk of tracheal damage. A plastic cuffed tube is disposable. The cuff and the tube won't separate inside the trachea because the cuff is bonded to the tube; it doesn't require periodic deflating to lower pressure because cuff pressure is low and evenly distributed against the tracheal wall, and it reduces the risk of tracheal damage. A plastic fenestrated tube permits speech through the upper airway when the external opening is capped and the cuff is deflated. It also allows easy removal of the inner cannula for cleaning, but it may become occluded.

CONTRAINDICATIONS
None known.

EQUIPMENT
For aseptic stoma and outer-cannula care
Waterproof trash bag ● two sterile solution containers ● sterile normal saline solution ● hydrogen peroxide ● sterile cotton-tipped applicators ● sterile 4″ × 4″ gauze pads ● sterile gloves ● prepackaged sterile tracheostomy dressing (or drain sponge) ● supplies for suctioning and mouth care ● water-soluble lubricant or topical antibiotic cream ● materials for cuff procedures and changing tracheostomy ties

For aseptic inner-cannula care
All preceding equipment plus a prepackaged commercial tracheostomy care set, or sterile forceps ● sterile nylon brush ● sterile 6″ (15-cm) pipe cleaners ● clean gloves ● a third sterile solution container ● disposable temporary inner cannula

For changing tracheostomy ties
30″ (76.2-cm) length of tracheostomy twill tape ● bandage scissors ● sterile gloves ● hemostat

For emergency tracheostomy tube replacement
RED FLAG The following supplies should always be kept at the bedside of a patient with a tracheostomy tube.
Sterile tracheal dilator or sterile hemostat ● sterile obturator that fits the tracheostomy tube ● an extra sterile tracheostomy tube that's the same size as the tube the patient has in place and one a size smaller, each with its packaged obturator ● suction equipment and supplies

For cuff procedures
5- or 10-ml syringe ● padded hemostat ● stethoscope

PREPARATION OF EQUIPMENT
■ Make sure there's a handheld resuscitation bag with the appropriate adapter and a face mask (in case of accidental decannulation) at the bedside.
■ Wash your hands and assemble equipment and supplies in the patient's room.
■ Check the expiration date on each sterile package and inspect for tears.
■ Establish a sterile field near the patient's bed and place equipment and supplies on it.
■ Place the open waterproof trash bag next to you to avoid reaching across the sterile field or the patient's stoma when discarding soiled items.
■ Pour normal saline solution, hydrogen peroxide, or a mixture of equal parts of both solutions into one of the sterile solution containers; pour normal saline solution into the second sterile container for rinsing.
■ For inner-cannula care, use a third sterile solution container to hold the gauze pads and cotton-tipped applicators saturated with cleaning solution.
■ If replacing the disposable inner cannula, open the package containing the new inner cannula while maintaining sterile technique.
■ Obtain or prepare new tracheostomy ties, if indicated.
■ Keep supplies in full view for easy emergency access.

ESSENTIAL STEPS
■ Reinforce the explanation of the procedure to the patient.

- Provide privacy.
- Place the patient in semi-Fowler's position, unless contraindicated, to decrease abdominal pressure on the diaphragm and promote lung expansion.
- Remove humidification, supplemental oxygen, or ventilation device.
- Using sterile technique, suction the entire length of the tracheostomy tube to clear the airway of secretions that may hinder oxygenation.
- Reconnect the patient to the humidifier, supplemental oxygen, or ventilator, if necessary.

Cleaning a stoma and outer cannula

- Put on sterile gloves.
- With your dominant hand, saturate a sterile gauze pad or cotton-tipped applicator with half-strength peroxide with normal saline or the prescribed cleaning solution.
- Squeeze out excess liquid to prevent accidental aspiration.
- Steady the tracheostomy tube with the nonsterile hand to prevent movement and discomfort to the patient.
- Wipe the patient's neck under the tracheostomy tube flanges and twill tapes.
- Saturate a second pad or applicator and clean the skin surrounding the tracheostomy. Use additional pads or cotton-tipped applicators to clean the stoma site and the tube's flanges.

RED FLAG Wipe only once with each pad or applicator to prevent contamination of a clean area.

- Rinse debris and peroxide (if used) with one or more sterile 4″ × 4″ gauze pads dampened in normal saline solution.
- Dry the area thoroughly with additional sterile gauze pads; then apply a new sterile tracheostomy dressing.
- Remove and discard your gloves.

Cleaning a nondisposable inner cannula

- Put on sterile gloves. Using your nondominant hand, remove and discard the patient's tracheostomy dressing.
- With the same hand, disconnect the ventilator or humidification device, and unlock the tracheostomy tube's inner cannula by rotating it counterclockwise.
- Place the inner cannula in the container of hydrogen peroxide.
- Working quickly, use your dominant hand to scrub the cannula with the sterile nylon brush.
- If the brush doesn't slide easily into the cannula, use a sterile pipe cleaner.

🚩 **RED FLAG** *Avoid scratching or damaging the inner cannula. Damaged areas can harbor bacteria.*

■ Immerse the cannula in the container of normal saline solution and agitate it for about 10 seconds to rinse it.

■ Inspect the cannula for cleanliness. Repeat the cleaning process if necessary.

■ If the cannula is clean, tap it against the inside edge of the sterile container to remove excess liquid and prevent aspiration.

🚩 **RED FLAG** *Don't dry the outer surface; a film of moisture acts as a lubricant during insertion.*

■ Reinsert the inner cannula into the patient's tracheostomy tube.

■ Lock it in place and make sure it's positioned securely. Reconnect the mechanical ventilator. Apply a new sterile tracheostomy dressing.

■ If the patient can't tolerate being disconnected from the ventilator for the time it takes to clean the inner cannula, replace the existing inner cannula with a clean one and reattach the mechanical ventilator. Clean the cannula you removed and store it in a sterile container for later use.

Caring for a disposable inner cannula

■ Put on clean gloves. Using your dominant hand, remove the inner cannula.

■ After evaluating the secretions in the cannula, discard it properly.

■ Pick up the new inner cannula, touching only the outer locking portion. Insert the cannula into the tracheostomy and, following manufacturer's instructions, lock it securely.

Changing tracheostomy ties

■ Get help from another nurse or a respiratory therapist to avoid accidental tube expulsion. If an assistant isn't available, the new ties can be fastened before the old ones are removed. Patient movement or coughing can dislodge the tube.

■ Wash your hands and put on sterile gloves.

■ If you aren't using commercially packaged tracheostomy ties, prepare new ties from a 30″ (76.2 cm) length of twill tape by folding one end back 1″ (2.5 cm) onto itself; then, with bandage scissors, cut a ½″ (1.3-cm) slit down the center of the tape from the folded edge.

■ Prepare the other end of the tape the same way.

■ Hold both ends together and cut the resulting circle of tape so one piece is about 10″ (25.5 cm) long and the other is about 20″ (51 cm) long.

■ Assist the patient into semi-Fowler's position, if possible.

■ Have your assistant put on gloves, and instruct her to hold the tracheostomy tube in place to prevent expulsion during replacement of the ties. (If performing without assistance, fasten the clean ties in place before removing the old ties to prevent tube expulsion.)

■ While the assistant's gloved fingers hold the tracheostomy tube in place, cut the soiled tracheostomy ties with bandage scissors, or untie them, and discard.

▶ *RED FLAG When you're cutting tracheostomy ties, be careful not to cut the tube of the pilot balloon.*

■ Thread the slit end of one new tie a short distance through the eye of one tracheostomy tube flange from the underside; use the hemostat, if needed, to pull the tie through. Thread the other end of the tie completely through the slit end and pull it taut so it loops firmly through the flange. This avoids knots that can cause throat discomfort, tissue irritation, pressure, and necrosis.

■ Fasten the second tie to the opposite flange in the same manner.

■ Instruct the patient to flex his neck while you bring the ties around to the side; tie them together with a square knot. Flexion produces the same neck circumference as coughing and helps prevent an overly tight tie.

■ Have your assistant place one finger under the tapes as you tie them to ensure they're tight enough to avoid slippage but loose enough to prevent choking, jugular vein constriction, or skin breakdown.

▶ *RED FLAG Be especially careful that tracheostomy ties aren't too tight on the patient with increased intracranial pressure; tight tracheostomy ties can further increase the pressure.*

■ Placing the closure on the side allows easy access and prevents pressure necrosis at the back of the neck when the patient is recumbent.

■ After securing the ties, cut off excess tape with scissors and have your assistant release the tracheostomy tube.

■ Make sure the patient is comfortable and can reach the call bell easily.

▶ *RED FLAG Check tracheostomy-tie tension frequently on patients with traumatic injury, radical neck dissection, or cardiac failure because neck diameter can increase from swelling and cause constriction. Check the ties on a restless patient to ensure ties don't come loose.*

Concluding tracheostomy care
■ Replace humidification or supplemental oxygen.
■ Provide oral care as needed because the oral cavity can become dry and malodorous or develop sores from encrusted secretions. Oral care should be performed every 2 hours and as needed.
■ Observe soiled dressings and suctioned secretions for amount, color, consistency, and odor. Properly clean or dispose of equipment, supplies, solutions, and trash. Remove and discard your gloves.
■ Make sure the patient is comfortable and can reach the call bell easily.
■ Make sure necessary supplies are readily available at the bedside.
■ Repeat the procedure at least once every 8 hours, according to the physician's orders, or as needed.
■ Change the dressing as often as necessary regardless of whether you perform the entire cleaning procedure. A wet dressing with exudate or secretions predisposes the patient to skin excoriation, breakdown, and infection.

Deflating and inflating a tracheostomy cuff
■ Read the cuff manufacturer's instructions because cuff types and procedures vary.
■ Monitor the patient's condition, reinforce the explanation of the procedure, and reassure him.
■ Wash your hands.
■ Help the patient into semi-Fowler's position, if possible, or place him in a supine position so secretions above the cuff site will be pushed up into his mouth if he's receiving positive-pressure ventilation.
■ Suction the oropharyngeal cavity to prevent pooled secretions from descending into the trachea after cuff deflation.
■ Release the padded hemostat clamping the cuff inflation tubing if a hemostat is present.
■ Insert a 5- or 10-ml syringe into the cuff pilot balloon and slowly withdraw all air from the cuff. Leave the syringe attached to tubing for cuff reinflation.
■ Slow deflation allows positive lung pressure to push secretions upward from the bronchi. Cuff deflation may also stimulate the cough reflex, producing additional secretions.
■ Remove the ventilation device and suction the lower airway through the existing tube to remove all secretions.
■ Reconnect the patient to the ventilation device.
■ Maintain cuff deflation for the prescribed time.

■ Observe for adequate ventilation and suction as necessary.

■ If the patient has difficulty breathing, reinflate the cuff immediately by depressing the syringe plunger slowly.

■ Use a stethoscope to listen over the trachea for the air leak, then inject as little air as necessary to achieve an adequate tracheal seal.

■ When inflating the cuff you may use the minimal-leak technique or the minimal occlusive volume technique to help gauge the proper inflation point.

■ If inflating the cuff using cuff pressure measurement, don't exceed 25 mm Hg.

RED FLAG Recommended cuff pressure is about 18 mm Hg. If pressure exceeds 25 mm Hg, notify the physician. You may need to change to a larger tube, use higher inflation pressures, or permit a larger air leak.

■ After you have inflated the cuff, if the tubing doesn't have a one-way valve at the end, clamp the inflation line with a padded hemostat and remove the syringe.

■ Check for a minimal-leak cuff seal. You shouldn't feel air coming from the patient's mouth, nose, or tracheostomy site, and a conscious patient shouldn't be able to speak.

■ Be alert for air leaks from the cuff itself.

RED FLAG Suspect a leak if injection of air fails to inflate the cuff or increase cuff pressure if you can't inject the amount of air you withdrew, if the patient can speak, if ventilation fails to maintain adequate respiratory movement with pressures or volumes previously considered adequate, or if air escapes during the ventilator's inspiratory cycle.

■ Make sure the patient is comfortable and can easily reach the call bell and communication aids.

■ Properly clean or dispose of equipment, supplies, and trash according to your facility's policy.

■ Replenish used supplies and make sure all necessary emergency supplies are at the bedside.

SPECIAL CONSIDERATIONS

■ Keep appropriate equipment at the patient's bedside for immediate use in an emergency.

RED FLAG Follow your facility's policy if a tracheostomy tube is expelled or the outer cannula becomes blocked. If breathing is obstructed, call the appropriate code and provide manual resuscitation with a handheld resuscitation bag and mask. Don't remove the tracheostomy tube; the airway may close completely. Use caution when reinserting the tube to avoid tracheal trauma, perforation, compression, and asphyxiation.

■ Don't change tracheostomy ties unnecessarily during the immediate postoperative period before the stoma track is well formed (usually 4 days) to avoid accidental dislodgment and expulsion of the tube. Unless secretions or drainage is a problem, ties can be changed once per day.

■ Don't change a single-cannula tracheostomy tube or the outer cannula of a double-cannula tube. Because of the risk of tracheal complications, the physician usually changes these kinds of cannulas; the frequency depends on the patient's condition and the condition of the cannula.

■ If the patient's neck or stoma is excoriated or infected, apply a water-soluble lubricant or topical antibiotic cream, as ordered. Don't use a powder or oil-based substance on or around a stoma; aspiration can cause infection and abscess.

■ Replace all equipment regularly (including solutions) to reduce the risk of nosocomial infections.

■ Reinforce the explanation of the procedure even if the patient is unresponsive.

■ Confirm the patient's diet order. Many patients with tracheostomy tubes are maintained on nothing-by-mouth because the risk for aspiration is high.

■ If the patient will be discharged with a tracheostomy, reinforce self-care teaching continuously.

■ Reinforce patient teaching about how to change and clean the tube.

■ If the patient is being discharged with suction equipment, make sure he and his family are knowledgeable and comfortable about using the equipment and make sure the patient has all the necessary home care and equipment referrals, if necessary.

COMPLICATIONS

Hemorrhage at operative site can cause drowning. Bleeding or edema in tracheal tissue may cause airway obstruction. The patient may aspirate his secretions. Air can be introduced into the pleural cavity causing pneumothorax. Hypoxia or acidosis can trigger cardiac arrest. Introduction of air into surrounding tissues causes subcutaneous emphysema. Secretions under dressings and twill tape can cause skin excoriation and infection. Hardened mucus or a slipped cuff can occlude the cannula opening and obstruct the patient's airway. Tube displacement can stimulate cough reflex if the tip rests on the carina, or it can cause blood vessel erosion and hemorrhage. Tracheal erosion and necrosis can occur.

DOCUMENTATION

■ Record the date, time, and type of procedure.

■ Note the amount, consistency, color, and odor of secretions.

■ Document the stoma, skin condition around the stoma, and care provided.

■ Record the patient's respiratory status.

■ Note the change of the tracheostomy tube by the physician.

■ Record the duration of cuff deflation and the amount of air used for cuff inflation.

■ Record cuff pressure readings and specific body position.

■ Note any complications and nursing actions taken.

■ Document the patient's or family's response to reinforced teaching.

■ Record the patient's tolerance of the treatment.

6

NEUROMUSCULAR CARE

The goals of neuromuscular care are to preserve and restore optimal nervous and musculoskeletal system function and prevent further deterioration or complications. Precise nursing skills and meticulous attention to detail are indispensable to achieving effective care.

Bone marrow aspiration and biopsy assistance

A specimen of bone marrow—the major site of blood cell formation—may be obtained by aspiration or needle biopsy. Aspiration removes cells through a needle inserted into the marrow cavity of the bone. A biopsy removes a small, solid core of marrow tissue through the needle. Both procedures are usually performed by a physician, but some trained chemotherapy nurses or nurse clinicians perform them with assistance. The procedure allows evaluation of overall blood composition by studying blood elements and precursor cells as well as abnormal or malignant cells. Aspirates aid in diagnosing various disorders and cancers, such as oat cell carcinoma, leukemia, and lymphomas such as Hodgkin's disease. Biopsies are commonly performed simultaneously to stage the disease and monitor response to treatment.

CONTRAINDICATIONS
None known.

EQUIPMENT
For aspiration
Prepackaged bone marrow set, which includes povidone-iodine pads • two sterile drapes (one fenestrated, one plain) • ten 4″ × 4″ gauze pads • ten 2″ × 2″ gauze pads • two 12-ml syringes • 22G 1″ or 2″ needle • scalpel • sedative • specimen containers • bone

marrow needle ● 70% isopropyl alcohol ● 1% lidocaine (unopened bottle) ● 26G or 27G ½″ to ⅝″ needle ● adhesive tape ● sterile gloves ● glass slides and cover glass labels

For biopsy
All equipment listed above ● Vim-Silverman, Jamshidi, Illinois sternal, or Westerman-Jensen needle ● Zenker's fixative

PREPARATION OF EQUIPMENT
■ Check for sterility and the expiration date of the prepackaged tray.
■ Assemble the equipment at the patient's bedside.

ESSENTIAL STEPS
■ Verify the patient's identity using two patient identifiers, such as the patient's name and identification number.
■ Make sure an informed consent form has been signed.
■ Check the patient's history for hypersensitivity to the local anesthetic and iodine or shellfish.
■ Provide an oral sedative (or have the registered nurse give an I.V. sedative) before the test, if ordered.
■ Position the patient appropriately for the selected puncture site. (See *Common sites for bone marrow aspiration and biopsy*.)
■ The team should take a "time out" to make sure that the right procedure is being performed on the right patient at the right site.
■ Assist the physician to clean the puncture site with povidone-iodine solution using sterile technique.
■ Allow the site to dry and help the physician drape the area.
■ To anesthetize the site, the physician infiltrates it with 1% lidocaine using a 26G or 27G ½″ to ⅝″ needle to inject a small amount intradermally, then a larger 22G 1″ to 2″ needle to anesthetize the tissue down to the bone.
■ When the needle tip reaches the bone, the physician anesthetizes the periosteum by injecting a small amount of lidocaine in a circular area about ¾″ (2 cm) in diameter.
■ The needle should be withdrawn from the periosteum after each injection.
■ After about 1 minute is allowed for the lidocaine to take effect, a scalpel may be used to make a small stab incision in the patient's skin to accommodate the bone marrow needle. This technique avoids pushing skin into the bone marrow, helps avoid unnecessary skin tearing, and reduces the risk of infection.

Common sites for bone marrow aspiration and biopsy

The posterior superior iliac crest is the preferred site for aspiration because no vital organs or vessels are nearby. The patient is placed in either a lateral position with one leg flexed or in a prone position.

For aspiration or biopsy from the anterior iliac crest, the patient is placed in the supine or side-lying position. This site is used with patients who can't lie prone because of severe abdominal distention.

Aspiration from the sternum involves the greatest risk but may be chosen because the site is near the surface, the cortical bone is thin, and the marrow cavity contains numerous cells and relatively little fat or supporting bone. The sternum is seldom used for biopsy.

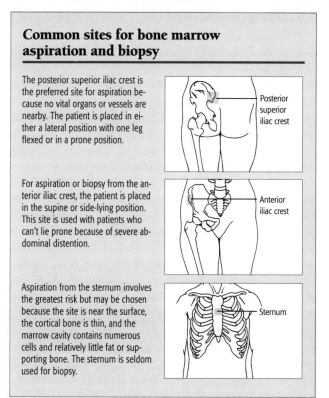

Bone marrow aspiration
- The physician inserts the bone marrow needle and lodges it firmly in the bone cortex.
- If the patient feels sharp pain instead of pressure when the needle first touches bone, the needle was probably inserted outside the anesthetized area.
- To correct the needle insertion, the physician withdraws slightly and moves toward the anesthetized area.
- The needle is advanced by applying an even, downward force with the heel of the hand or the palm, while twisting it back and forth slightly.

■ A crackling sensation means the needle has entered the marrow cavity.
■ The physician removes the inner cannula, attaches the syringe to the needle, aspirates the required specimen, and withdraws the needle.
■ The specimen is placed on glass slides and covered with the coverglass.
■ Label the specimen with the patient's name and the date.
■ Put on gloves and apply pressure to the aspiration site with a gauze pad for 5 minutes to control bleeding, while an assistant prepares the marrow slides.
■ Clean the area with alcohol to remove the povidone-iodine.
■ Dry the skin thoroughly with a 4″ × 4″ gauze pad, and apply a sterile pressure dressing.

Bone marrow biopsy
■ The physician inserts the biopsy needle into the periosteum and advances it steadily until the outer needle passes into the marrow cavity.
■ The biopsy needle is directed into the marrow cavity by alternately rotating the inner needle clockwise and counterclockwise.
■ A plug of tissue is removed, the needle assembly is withdrawn, and the marrow specimen is expelled into a properly labeled specimen bottle containing Zenker's fixative or formaldehyde.
■ Put on gloves.
■ Clean the area around the biopsy site with alcohol to remove the povidone-iodine solution.
■ Firmly press a sterile 2″ × 2″ gauze pad against the incision to control bleeding and apply a sterile pressure dressing.
■ If a hematoma occurs around the puncture site, apply warm soaks and give analgesics for site pain or tenderness.

SPECIAL CONSIDERATIONS
■ Faulty needle placement may yield too little aspirate.
■ If no specimen is produced, the needle must be withdrawn from the bone (but not from the overlying soft tissue), the stylet replaced, and the needle inserted into a second site within the anesthetized field.
■ Bone marrow specimens shouldn't be collected from irradiated areas because radiation may have altered or destroyed the marrow.
■ Reinforce the explanation of the procedure to the patient to ease anxiety and ensure cooperation.

■ Make sure the patient or a responsible family member understands the procedure and signs a consent form.
■ Remind the patient that the procedure usually takes 5 to 10 minutes, test results are usually available in one day, and more than one marrow specimen may be required.
■ Remind the patient which bone will be sampled.
■ Tell the patient that he'll receive a local anesthetic.
■ Reinforce that he'll feel heavy pressure from insertion of the biopsy or aspiration needle, as well as a brief, pulling sensation.
■ Remind the patient that the physician may make a small incision to avoid tearing the skin.
■ If the patient has osteoporosis, explain that the needle pressure may be minimal and that a drill may be needed.

COMPLICATIONS

Potential complications include puncturing the heart and major vessels, causing severe hemorrhage; puncturing the mediastinum, causing mediastinitis or pneumomediastinum; and puncturing the lung, causing pneumothorax.

 ***RED FLAG** Bleeding and infection are potentially life-threatening complications of aspiration or biopsy at any site.*

DOCUMENTATION

■ Document the time, date, location, and patient's tolerance of the procedure and what specimen was obtained.
■ Document a description of the puncture site and the amount of time pressure was held.

Cast application

Casts are hard molds that encase a body part, usually an extremity, to provide immobilization of bones and surrounding tissue. They can be used to treat injuries (including fractures), correct orthopedic conditions (such as deformities), or promote healing after general or plastic surgery, amputation, or nerve and vascular repair. They may be constructed of fiberglass or other synthetic materials. Fiberglass is lighter, stronger, and more resilient than plaster, but it's more difficult to mold because it dries rapidly. It can bear body weight immediately, if necessary. (See *Types of cylindrical casts,* page 154.)

A physician usually applies a cast; the nurse prepares the patient and equipment and assists with the procedure.

Types of cylindrical casts

Made of fiberglass or other synthetic materials, casts may be applied almost anywhere on the body to support a single finger or the entire body. Common casts are shown here.

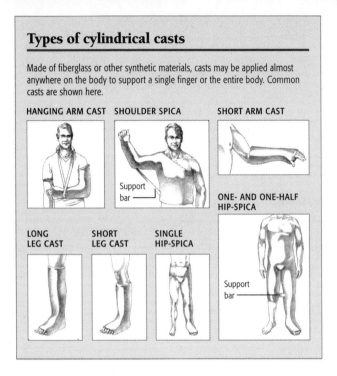

HANGING ARM CAST   **SHOULDER SPICA**   **SHORT ARM CAST**

Support bar

ONE- AND ONE-HALF HIP-SPICA

LONG LEG CAST   **SHORT LEG CAST**   **SINGLE HIP-SPICA**

Support bar

CONTRAINDICATIONS
- Skin diseases
- Peripheral vascular disease
- Diabetes mellitus
- Open or draining wounds
- Overwhelming edema
- Susceptibility to skin irritations

EQUIPMENT
Casting material ● plaster rolls ● tubular stockinette ● plaster splints (if necessary) ● bucket of water ● sink equipped with plaster trap ● linen-saver pad ● sheet ● wadding ● sponge or felt padding (if necessary)

PREPARATION OF EQUIPMENT

■ Gently squeeze packaged casting material to make sure envelopes don't have air leaks.

■ Room temperature or slightly warmer water is best because it allows the cast to set in about 7 minutes without excessive exothermia.

■ Cold water slows the rate of setting and may be used to facilitate difficult molding.

■ Warm water speeds the rate of setting and raises skin temperature under the cast.

ESSENTIAL STEPS

■ Verify the patient's identity using two patient identifiers, such as the patient's name and identification number.

■ Reinforce the explanation of the procedure to allay patient's fears and support informed consent.

■ Cover the patient's bedding and gown with a linen-saver pad.

■ If the cast is applied to a wrist or arm, remove the patient's rings and bracelets to prevent circulation problems.

■ Check the condition of the patient's skin in the affected area, noting redness, contusions, or open wounds, to aid in evaluating complaints he may have after the cast is applied.

■ If the patient has an open wound, prepare him for a local anesthetic.

■ Clean the wound.

■ Assist the physician as he closes the wound and applies a dressing.

■ Monitor the patient's neurovascular status by palpating the distal pulses and monitoring color, temperature, and capillary refill of appropriate fingers or toes.

■ Monitor neurologic function, including sensation and motion in extremities.

■ If possible, wash and dry the patient's skin.

■ Help the physician to position the limb. The limb is usually immobilized in a neutral position.

■ Support the limb in the prescribed position while the physician applies the tubular stockinette and sheet wadding. The stockinette, if used, should extend past the cast's ends to pad the edges.

Preparing a cotton and polyester cast

■ Assist the physician to immerse the roll in cold water. Squeeze it four times to ensure uniform wetness.

RED FLAG *Open casting materials one roll at a time because cotton and polyester casting must be applied within 3 minutes—before humidity in the air hardens the tape.*

■ Remove the dripping wet material from the bucket.
■ Remind the patient that the material will feel warm, giving off heat as it sets.

Preparing a fiberglass cast

■ If a water-activated fiberglass material is used, assist the physician to immerse the tape rolls in tepid water for 10 to 15 minutes to start the chemical reaction that causes the cast to harden.
■ Open one roll at a time.

RED FLAG *Excess water shouldn't be squeezed out before application.*

■ If the physician is using light-cured fiberglass, he'll unroll the material more slowly.
■ Light-cured fiberglass casting remains soft and malleable until it's exposed to ultraviolet light, which sets it.

Completing the cast

■ As necessary, work with the physician to "petal" the cast's edges to reduce roughness and cushion pressure points. (See *How to petal a cast*.)
■ Assist the physician by using a cast stand or your palm to support the cast in the therapeutic position until it becomes firm (6 to 8 minutes) to prevent indentations. (This is especially important with a plaster cast.)
■ The cast will be placed on a firm, smooth surface to continue drying.
■ Help place pillows under joints to maintain flexion, if necessary.
■ Monitor circulation in the casted limb by palpating the distal pulse, and monitor color, temperature, and capillary refill of fingers or toes.
■ Monitor neurologic status by asking the patient if he's experiencing paresthesia in the extremity or decreased motion of the extremity's uncovered joints.
■ Monitor the unaffected extremity and compare findings.
■ Elevate the limb above heart level with pillows or bath blankets to facilitate venous return and reduce edema.
■ The physician will send the patient for X-rays to ensure proper positioning.

How to petal a cast

Rough cast edges can be cushioned by petaling them with adhesive tape or moleskin. To do this, cut several 4" × 2" (10- × 5-cm) strips. Round off one end of each strip to keep it from curling. Then making sure the rounded end of the strip is on the outside of the cast, tuck the straight end just inside the cast edge (as shown).

Smooth the moleskin with your finger until you're sure it's secured inside and out. Repeat the procedure, overlapping the moleskin pieces until you've covered the cast's edge (as shown)

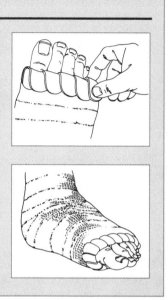

SPECIAL CONSIDERATIONS

■ A fiberglass cast dries immediately after application.
■ During the drying period, the cast must be properly positioned to prevent a surface depression that could cause pressure areas or dependent edema.
■ Never use the bed or a table to support the cast as it sets because molding can result, causing pressure necrosis of underlying tissue.
■ Don't use rubber- or plastic-covered pillows before the cast hardens because they can trap heat under the cast.
■ Avoid using hair dryers or fans to speed drying because uneven drying can occur.
■ After the cast dries completely, it no longer feels damp or soft.
■ Care consists of monitoring the patient for changes in drainage pattern, neurovascular status, and the condition of the cast; preventing skin breakdown near the cast; and assisting the patient to deal with immobility.

- Start patient teaching right after the cast is applied and continue it until the patient or a family member can care for the cast.
- If a cast is applied after surgery or traumatic injury, the most accurate way to monitor the patient for bleeding is to track and compare vital signs.

  RED FLAG *A visible blood spot on the cast can be misleading: One drop of blood can produce a circle 3" (7.6 cm) in diameter.*

- Casts may need to be opened to monitor underlying skin or pulses or to relieve pressure in a specific area.
- In a windowed cast, an area is cut out to allow inspection of skin or relieve pressure.
- A bivalved cast is split medially and laterally, creating anterior and posterior sections, and one section may be removed to relieve pressure while the other maintains immobilization.
- Reinforce that the patient needs to keep the limb above heart level to minimize swelling.
- Elevate a leg by having the patient lie down with his leg propped on pillows.
- Prop a casted arm so the hand and elbow are higher than the shoulder.

  RED FLAG *Remind the patient to call the physician if he can't move his fingers or toes, if he has numbness or tingling or loss of sensation in the affected limb, or has symptoms of infection such as fever, unusual pain, or a foul odor from the cast.*

- Reinforce that the patient can help maintain some muscle strength by doing recommended exercises.
- If the cast needs repair or if the patient has questions about cast care, remind him to notify his physician.
- Remind the patient to keep the cast from getting wet because moisture will weaken or ruin it.
- If the physician approves, have the patient cover the cast with a plastic bag or cast cover for showering or bathing.
- Reinforce that the patient shouldn't insert anything into the cast to relieve itching because foreign matter can damage skin and cause infection. He can use alcohol on the skin at the cast edges.

  RED FLAG *Reinforce that patient shouldn't chip, crush, cut, or otherwise break any area of the cast. He should not bear weight on the cast unless told to do so by the physician.*

- If the patient must use crutches, remind him to remove throw rugs and rearrange furniture to reduce risk of tripping.
- If he has a cast on his dominant arm, the patient may need help from an occupational therapist to learn ways to facilitate bathing, using the toilet, eating, and dressing.

- The physician removes the cast at the appropriate time, with a nurse assisting.
- Muscle atrophy and skin flaking are expected results of casting. Reinforce with the patient that when the cast is removed, the limb will appear thinner than the uncasted limb and the skin will appear yellowish or gray. Remind the patient that exercise and skin care will return muscle atrophy and skin color to normal.

COMPLICATIONS

Complications of casting include compartment syndrome, palsy, paresthesia, ischemia, ischemic myositis, pressure necrosis, misalignment or nonunion of fractured bones, and skin breakdown.

DOCUMENTATION

- Document the date and time of application and the patient's skin condition before cast was applied.
- Note any contusions, redness, or open wounds.
- Record any results of neurovascular checks, before and after application, for affected and unaffected limbs.
- Describe the location of special devices, such as felt pads or plaster splints.
- Document the type of cast applied.
- Note patient teaching.

Fall prevention and management

Falls can occur because of poor lighting, slippery floors, throw rugs, unfamiliar surroundings, or physiologic factors, such as confusion, agitation, temporary muscle paralysis, vertigo, orthostatic hypotension, central nervous system lesions, dementia, failing eyesight, and decreased strength or coordination. With elderly patients, fall injuries can cause psychological problems, loss of self-confidence, and fear, and they can hasten a move to a long-term care facility.

CONTRAINDICATIONS

None known.

EQUIPMENT

Stethoscope ● sphygmomanometer ● analgesics ● cold and warm compresses ● pillows ● blankets ● emergency resuscitation equipment (crash cart), if needed ● electrocardiograph (ECG) monitor, if needed

PREPARATION OF EQUIPMENT

■ If helping a fallen patient, send someone for monitoring or resuscitation equipment.

ESSENTIAL STEPS

■ Use patience and caution whether your care plan focuses on preventing falls or managing one in an elderly patient.

■ The registered nurse should assess the patient's risk for falling on admission, or according to your facility's policy. Periodic reassessment should take place when the patient's condition changes, when he's moved to another level of care, or when medications are prescribed that increase his risk for falling.

Preventing falls

■ Monitor patient's fall risk at least once each shift (at least every 3 months if patient is in a long-term care facility). Your facility may require more frequent monitoring. Note any changes in his condition that increase the risk of falling, such as confusion and mobility issues.

■ If the patient is at risk, take steps to ensure his safety and correct potential dangers in his environment.

■ Position the call bell so the patient can reach it.

■ Provide adequate nighttime lighting.

■ Place the patient's personal belongings, assistive devices, care aids, the telephone, and his overbed table within easy reach.

■ Encourage patients with I.V. poles and other equipment to call for assistance when getting out of bed.

■ Instruct the patient to rise slowly from a supine position.

■ Keep the bed in its lowest position so the patient can reach the floor when he gets out of bed.

■ Lock the bed's wheels and place the bed against the wall, if possible.

■ Frequently check the patient if any of the side rails are in the raised position.

■ Advise the patient to wear nonskid footwear.

■ Check the patient at least every 2 hours.

■ Check a high-risk patient every 30 minutes.

■ If possible, keep high-risk patients near the nursing station so that they can be monitored closely.

■ If the patient is unable to make it to the bathroom quickly, place a commode at the bedside.

■ Empty all drains in a timely fashion to prevent leakage on the floor that may cause the patient to slip.

■ Implement a toileting regimen to prevent falls related to incontinence.
■ Alert other caregivers to the patient's risk for falling and to interventions you've implemented.
■ Encourage the patient to perform active range-of-motion exercises to improve his flexibility and coordination.

Managing falls

■ If you're with the patient as he falls, try to break his fall with your body.
■ As you guide the patient to the floor, support his body—particularly his head and trunk.
■ If possible, help the patient to a supine position.
■ Try to maintain proper body alignment yourself to keep the center of gravity within your support base. Spread your feet to widen your support base. The wider the base, the better your balance will be.
■ Bend your knees—not your back—to support the patient and avoid injuring yourself.
■ Remain calm and stay with the patient to prevent further injury.
■ Monitor the patient's airway, breathing, and circulation. Help determine if the fall was caused by respiratory or cardiac arrest. If you don't detect respirations or a pulse, initiate emergency resuscitation measures.
■ Note the patient's level of consciousness (LOC); monitor pupil size, equality, and reaction to light.
■ Check for injuries, such as lacerations, abrasions, and obvious deformities.
■ Take steps to control bleeding.
■ Note any deviations from the patient's baseline condition.
■ If you weren't present during the fall, ask the patient or a witness what happened. Ask if he experienced pain or a change in LOC.
■ Don't move him until a physician fully evaluates his status and orders that the patient may be moved.

RED FLAG *Spinal cord injuries from falls are rare, but if one occurred, any movement may cause irreversible spinal damage.*

■ After the physician orders that the patient may be moved, call for assistance to get the patient back to bed.

RED FLAG *Never try to lift a patient alone; you may injure yourself or the patient.*

■ Provide reassurance as needed, and monitor for such signs and symptoms as confusion, tremor, weakness, pain, and dizziness.
■ Monitor the patient's limb strength and motion.

■ While the patient lies on the floor awaiting the physician, offer pillows and blankets for comfort.

■ *RED FLAG If you suspect a spinal cord injury, don't place a pillow under his head.*

■ The physician may order an X-ray if he suspects a fracture.

■ Provide first aid for minor injuries.

■ Monitor the patient's status for the next 24 hours.

■ Even if the patient shows no signs of distress or has only minor injuries, monitor his vital signs every 15 minutes for 1 hour, every 30 minutes the next hour, then every hour for 2 hours or until his condition stabilizes. Notify the physician if you note change from the baseline.

■ Perform necessary pain relief measures. Give analgesics, and apply cold compresses the first 24 hours and warm compresses thereafter.

■ Monitor the patient's environment and risk of falling. Discuss why he fell and how he thinks it could have been prevented.

■ Help determine if drugs may have contributed to the fall.

■ Monitor gait disturbances or improper use of canes, crutches, or walker.

SPECIAL CONSIDERATIONS

■ After a fall, review the patient's medical history for other complications; if he hit his head, check whether he takes anticoagulants and is at greater risk for intracranial bleeding. Monitor him accordingly.

■ Follow your facility's fall prevention program.

■ For a high-risk patient, in place of restraints, consider using a pressure pad or another alarm that warns when the patient gets out of bed.

■ Place the patient on an "at risk" status according to the facility policy. This may involve placing a bright colored bracelet on the patient, marking his call light with a bright colored sticker, or placing a sign on the door of the patient's room. Add appropriate nursing orders to the Kardex and chart.

■ Ensure the patient's call bell is answered promptly.

■ Provide emotional support during prevention and management of a fall.

■ Let the elderly patient know you recognize his limitations and acknowledge his fears. Point out measures that you'll take to provide a safe environment.

■ Reinforce with the patient how to fall safely.

■ If the patient uses a walker or a wheelchair, reinforce a demonstration of how to cope with and recover from a fall.

- Remind the patient to look for a low, sturdy, supportive piece of furniture to help himself up with; review the proper procedure for lifting himself and standing up with the walker or getting into the wheelchair.
- Before discharge, reinforce instructions to prevent accidental falls at home with the patient and family members.
- As needed, help refer the patient to the local visiting nurse association so nursing services can continue after discharge and during convalescence.

COMPLICATIONS
None known.

DOCUMENTATION
- Complete a detailed incident report after a fall in case of legal action.
- This report is mainly for insurance purposes, not part of the patient's record. Send copies to the facility administrator, who may evaluate care given in the unit and propose safety policies and performance improvement plans as appropriate.
- If the patient can recall what happened, quote the patient's description of the event.
- Note where and when the fall occurred, how the patient was found, and in what position.
- Record his vital signs.
- Document the events preceding the fall, names of witnesses, the patient's reaction to the fall, and a detailed description of his condition.
- Note interventions taken and the names of staff members who helped care for the patient after the fall.
- Record the physician's name and date and time he was notified; include a copy of the physician's report.
- Note if the patient was given diagnostic tests or transferred to another unit because of the fall.
- Note if the patient was monitored for a severe complication.

Lumbar puncture

Lumbar puncture involves insertion of a sterile needle into the subarachnoid space of the spinal canal, usually between the third and fourth lumbar vertebrae. It's used to determine the presence of blood in cerebrospinal fluid (CSF), to obtain CSF specimens for laboratory analysis, to inject dyes for contrast in radiologic studies, to administer drugs or anesthetics, and to relieve increased intracranial pressure (ICP) by removing CSF.

CONTRAINDICATIONS

■ Increased ICP
■ Lumbar deformity
■ Infection at the puncture site

EQUIPMENT

Overbed table ● a lumbar puncture kit or, if not available, ● two or three pairs of sterile gloves ● povidone-iodine solution ● sterile gauze pads ● alcohol pads ● sterile fenestrated drape ● 3-ml syringe for local anesthetic ● 25G ¾″ sterile needle for injecting anesthetic ● local anesthetic (usually 1% lidocaine) ● 18G or 20G 3½″ spinal needle with stylet (22G needle for children) ● three-way stopcock manometer ● small adhesive bandage ● three sterile collection tubes ● laboratory request forms ● labels ● patient-care reminder ● light source (optional)

PREPARATION OF EQUIPMENT

■ Gather the equipment and take it to the patient's bedside.
■ Check the sterility of the prepackaged tray and the expiration date.

ESSENTIAL STEPS

■ Verify the patient's identity using two patient identifiers, such as the patient's name and identification number.
■ Reinforce the explanation of the procedure to the patient to ease anxiety and ensure cooperation.
■ Make sure an informed consent form has been signed.
■ Provide privacy.
■ Instruct the patient to void immediately before the procedure.
■ Wash your hands.
■ Open the equipment tray on an overbed table using sterile technique.
■ Provide adequate lighting at the puncture site.
■ Adjust the bed height for physician comfort.
■ Position the patient and reemphasize the importance of remaining as still as possible to minimize discomfort and trauma. (See *Positioning for lumbar puncture.*)
■ The team should take a "time out" to verify that the right procedure is being done on the right patient at the right site.
■ Before the physician injects the anesthetic, reinforce with the patient that he'll experience a burning sensation and local pain. Ask

Positioning for lumbar puncture

Have the patient lie on his side at the edge of the bed, with his chin tucked to his chest and his knees drawn up to his abdomen. Make sure his spine is curved and his back is at the edge of the bed (as shown). This position widens the spaces between the vertebrae, easing needle insertion.

To help the patient maintain this position, place one of your hands behind his neck and the other hand behind his knees and pull gently. To prevent accidental needle displacement, hold the patient firmly in this position throughout the procedure.

Typically, the practitioner inserts the needle between the third and fourth lumbar vertebrae (as shown).

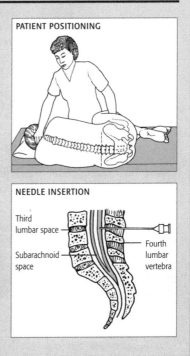

PATIENT POSITIONING

NEEDLE INSERTION

Third lumbar space

Subarachnoid space

Fourth lumbar vertebra

him to report any other persistent pain or sensations because this may indicate irritation or puncture of a nerve root, requiring repositioning of the needle.

■ The physician cleans the puncture site with sterile gauze pads soaked in povidone-iodine solution, wiping in a circular motion away from the puncture site.

■ The physician uses three different pads to prevent contamination of spinal tissues by the body's normal skin bacteria.

■ He drapes the area with the fenestrated drape to provide a sterile field. (If he uses povidone-iodine pads instead of sterile gauze pads, he may replace his sterile gloves to avoid introducing povidone-iodine into the subarachnoid space with the lumbar puncture needle.)

■ The physician anesthetizes the area. If the anesthetic isn't included on the equipment tray, clean the injection port of a multidose vial of anesthetic with an alcohol pad. Invert the vial 45 degrees so the physician can insert a 25G needle and syringe and withdraw anesthetic.

■ Remind the patient to remain still and breathe normally as the physician inserts the spinal needle.

■ Hold the patient firmly in position to prevent sudden movement.

■ If necessary, the physician attaches a manometer to the needle to read CSF pressure.

■ Help the patient extend his legs to provide an accurate reading.

■ If the physician suspects an obstruction in the spinal subarachnoid space, he may check for Queckenstedt's sign. After an initial CSF pressure reading, he compresses the patient's jugular vein for 10 seconds. This causes a rapid increase in ICP and causes CSF pressure to rise. When he takes pressure off the vein, the CSF pressure quickly returns to normal. If the vertebral canal is blocked, the CSF pressure doesn't vary, or only varies slightly, with the maneuver. The physician takes pressure readings every 10 seconds until pressure stabilizes.

■ The physician detaches the manometer and allows CSF to drain from the needle hub into the collection tubes, or injects dye or anesthetic if contrast media or spinal anesthetic is needed.

■ Mark the collection tubes in sequence (#1, #2, #3), secure their caps, and label them.

■ Put on sterile gloves.

■ After the spinal needle is removed, clean the puncture site with povidone-iodine and apply a small adhesive bandage.

■ Remove and discard gloves.

■ Send the CSF specimens to the laboratory immediately with a completed laboratory request form.

SPECIAL CONSIDERATIONS

■ Lumbar puncture is performed by a physician and requires sterile technique and careful patient positioning.

■ Watch closely for signs of adverse reaction: elevated pulse rate, pallor, and clammy skin. Alert the physician immediately of significant changes.

RED FLAG *The patient may be instructed to lie flat for 8 to 12 hours after the procedure. If necessary, place a patient-care reminder on his bed and keep his call bell in reach.*

■ Collected CSF specimens must be sent to the laboratory immediately.

■ Warn the patient that he may experience a headache after lumbar puncture. Reassure him that his cooperation during the procedure minimizes such an effect.

■ Reinforce the importance of remaining as still as possible to minimize discomfort and trauma.

COMPLICATIONS

Headache is the most common complication of a lumbar puncture. The patient can have a reaction to the anesthetic. He can develop meningitis, an epidural or subdural abscess, bleeding into the spinal canal, or CSF leakage from the puncture. Local pain may be caused by nerve root irritation. Edema or hematoma can develop at the puncture site. The patient may experience transient difficulty voiding after the test is completed. If infection occurs, he may also develop a fever.

RED FLAG The most serious complications of lumbar puncture, although rare, are tonsillar herniation and medullary compression.

DOCUMENTATION

■ Record the start and end times of the procedure.

■ Note the patient's response.

■ Document the administration of drugs.

■ Record the number of specimen tubes collected, the time of transport to the laboratory, and the color, consistency, and other characteristics of collected specimens.

■ Document the CSF pressures and the times they were obtained.

■ Document the amount of CSF drained.

Stump and prosthesis care

Patient care immediately after limb amputation includes monitoring drainage from the stump, positioning the affected limb, assisting with exercises prescribed by a physical therapist, and wrapping and conditioning the stump in preparation for prosthesis. Postoperative care will vary slightly, depending on the amputation site and whether an elastic bandage or plaster cast is used. After the stump heals, it requires only routine daily care (proper hygiene and continued muscle-strengthening exercises). A prosthesis must be cleaned and lubricated daily and checked for proper fit.

CONTRAINDICATIONS
None known.

EQUIPMENT
For postoperative stump care
Pressure dressing, abdominal pad ● suction equipment, if ordered ●
overhead trapeze ● 1″ adhesive tape ● bandage clips or safety pins ●
sandbags or trochanter roll (for a leg) ● elastic stump shrinker or 4″
elastic bandage ● tourniquet (optional, as last resort to control
bleeding)

For stump and prosthesis care
Mild soap ● stump socks or athletic tube socks ● two washcloths ●
two towels ● appropriate lubricating oil

ESSENTIAL STEPS
■ Perform routine postoperative care.
■ Make sure that the patient is comfortable, that his pain is man-
  aged, and that he's safe.

Monitoring stump drainage
■ Gravity causes fluid to accumulate at the stump. Frequently
  monitor the amount of blood and drainage on the dressing.
  *RED FLAG If accumulations of drainage or blood increase rapidly
  or excessive bleeding occurs, apply a pressure dressing or
  compress to the appropriate pressure points and notify the physician
  immediately.*
■ Tape the abdominal pad over the moist part of the dressing to
  provide a dry area to help prevent bacterial infection.
■ Monitor the suction drainage equipment, if present, and note the
  amount and type of drainage.

Positioning the extremity
■ Elevate the extremity above the heart for the first 24 hours.
■ To prevent contractures, position an arm with the elbow extended and the shoulder abducted.
■ To correctly position a leg, elevate the foot of the bed slightly and
  place sandbags or a trochanter roll against the hip to prevent external rotation.
  *RED FLAG Don't place a pillow under the thigh to flex the hip
  because this can cause hip flexion contracture. For the same
  reason, tell the patient to avoid prolonged sitting.*

■ After a below-the-knee amputation, maintain knee extension to prevent hamstring muscle contractures. Schedule four times during the day when the patient is purposefully in a supine position with his knee extended.

■ After a leg amputation, place the patient on a firm surface in the prone position for at least 2 hours per day, with his legs close together and without pillows under his abdomen, hips, knees, or stump, unless this position is contraindicated. If this position causes pain, the patient may require an analgesic as a premedication.

Assisting with prescribed exercises

■ After arm amputation, encourage the patient to exercise the remaining stump to prevent muscle contractures.

■ Help the patient perform isometric (muscles are flexed and held in a stationary position) and range-of-motion (ROM) exercises for both shoulders.

■ After leg amputation, stand behind the patient and, if necessary, support him with your hands at his waist during balancing exercises.

■ Remind the patient to exercise the affected and unaffected limbs to maintain muscle tone and increase muscle strength.

■ The patient with a leg amputation may perform push-ups in the sitting position, arms at his sides, or pull-ups on the overhead trapeze to strengthen his arms, shoulders, and back, in preparation for using crutches.

Wrapping and conditioning the stump

■ Apply an elastic stump shrinker to prevent edema and shape the limb in preparation for the prosthesis.

■ Wrap the stump so it narrows toward the distal end. This helps the prosthesis fit properly and ensures comfort when the patient wears it. (See *Wrapping a stump,* page 170.)

■ If an elastic stump shrinker isn't available you can wrap the stump in a 4″ elastic bandage. Stretch the bandage to about two-thirds its maximum length as you wrap it diagonally around the stump with the greatest pressure distally.

■ Make sure the bandage covers all portions of the stump smoothly because wrinkles or exposed areas can cause skin breakdown.

⚑ *RED FLAG If the patient experiences throbbing after the stump is wrapped, the bandage may be too tight. Remove the bandage immediately, reapply it slightly looser, and monitor it regularly.*

Wrapping a stump

Proper stump care helps protect the limb, reduces swelling, and prepares the limb for a prosthesis. As you perform the procedure, explain it to the patient.

Start by obtaining two 4" elastic bandages. Center the end of the first 4" bandage at the top of the patient's thigh. Unroll the bandage downward over the stump and to the back of the leg (as shown).

Make three figure-eight turns to adequately cover the ends of the stump. As you wrap, be sure to include the roll of flesh in the groin area. Use enough pressure to ensure that the stump narrows toward the end so that it fits comfortably into the prosthesis.

Use the second 4" bandage to anchor the first bandage around the waist. For a below-the-knee amputation, use the knee to anchor the bandage in place. Secure the bandage with clips, safety pins, or adhesive tape. Check the stump bandage regularly and rewrap it if it bunches at the end.

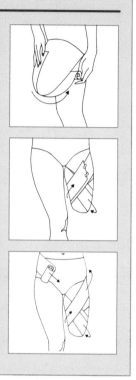

- Rewrap the bandage when it begins to bunch up at the end (typically about every 12 hours for a moderately active patient).
- After removing the bandage to rewrap it, massage the stump gently, always pushing toward the suture line rather than away from it.
- When healing begins, instruct the patient to push the stump against a pillow.
- Have the patient progress gradually to pushing against harder surfaces.

Caring for the healed stump

■ Bathe the stump at the end of the day. Be careful because warm water may cause swelling, making application of the prosthesis difficult. Don't soak the stump for long periods.

■ Don't apply lotion to the stump. This may clog hair follicles, increasing the risk of infection.

■ Avoid using powders or lotions, which can soften or irritate the skin.

■ Monitor the stump for redness, swelling, irritation, and calluses. Report these to the physician.

■ Change and wash the patient's elastic bandages every day to avoid exposing the skin to excessive perspiration.

■ To shape the stump, have the patient wear an elastic bandage 24 hours a day except while bathing.

■ To prevent infection, never shave the stump.

■ Tell the patient to avoid putting weight on the stump but to continue muscle-strengthening exercises.

Caring for the plastic prosthesis

■ Wipe the plastic socket of the prosthesis with a damp cloth and mild soap or alcohol to prevent bacterial accumulation.

■ Wipe the insert (if the prosthesis has one) with a dry cloth and dry the prosthesis thoroughly. When possible, allow it to dry overnight.

■ Maintain and lubricate the prosthesis and check for malfunctions.

■ Frequently monitor the condition of the shoe on a foot prosthesis and change it as necessary.

Applying the prosthesis

■ Apply a stump sock, keeping the seams away from bony prominences.

■ If the prosthesis has an insert, remove it from the socket, place it over the stump, and insert the stump into the prosthesis.

■ If it has no insert, slide the prosthesis over the stump.

■ Secure the prosthesis onto the stump according to the manufacturer's directions.

SPECIAL CONSIDERATIONS

■ If the patient arrives at the hospital with a traumatic amputation, the amputated part may be saved for possible reimplantation.

■ Exercise of the remaining muscles of an amputated limb must begin the day after surgery.

- Arm exercises progress from isometrics to assisted ROM to active ROM.
- Leg exercises include rising from a chair, balancing on one leg, and ROM exercises of the knees and hips.
- For a below-the-knee amputation, you may substitute an athletic tube sock for a stump sock by cutting off the elastic band.
- If the patient has a rigid dressing, perform normal cast care.
- If the cast slips off, apply an elastic bandage immediately and notify the physician because edema will develop rapidly.
- Reinforce teaching regarding how the patient should care for his stump and prosthesis.
- Encourage proper daily stump care and remind him that proper care of his stump can speed healing.
- Reinforce that the patient should inspect his stump every day, using a mirror.
- Remind the patient of the signs and symptoms that indicate problems in the stump.
- Remind the patient to call the physician if the incision appears to be opening, looks red or swollen, feels warm, is painful to touch, or is seeping drainage.
- Reinforce that a 10-lb (4.5-kg) change in body weight will alter his stump size and require a new prosthesis socket.
- Remind the patient to massage the stump toward the suture line to mobilize the scar and prevent its adherence to bone.
- Reinforce that the patient should avoid exposing the skin around the stump to excessive perspiration, which can cause irritation.
- Remind the patient to change his elastic bandages or stump socks daily.
- Reinforce that the patient may experience twitching, spasms, or phantom limb sensations (such as pain, warmth, cold, or itching) as his stump muscles adjust to amputation.
- Practice imagery, biofeedback, or distraction with the patient to relieve phantom limb pain or other sensations.
- Remind him to use mild heat, massage, or gentle pressure for these symptoms.
- If the patient's stump is sensitive to touch, reinforce that he should rub it with a dry washcloth for 4 minutes, three times a day.
- Reinforce the importance of performing prescribed exercises to help minimize complications, maintain muscle strength and tone, prevent contractures, and promote independence.
- Reinforce the importance of positioning to prevent contractures and edema.

COMPLICATIONS

Complications include hemorrhage, stump infection, contractures, a swollen or flabby stump, skin breakdown or irritation, friction from an irritant in the prosthesis, sebaceous cyst or boil, psychologic problems, and phantom limb pain.

DOCUMENTATION

■ Record the date, time, and specific procedures of postoperative care.
■ Note the amount and type of drainage and condition of the dressing.
■ Document the need for dressing reinforcement.
■ Record the appearance and condition of the suture line and surrounding tissue.
■ Note the patient's pain levels and analgesics given.
■ Record any signs of skin irritation or infection, such as redness or tenderness.
■ Record complications and nursing actions taken.
■ Note the patient's tolerance of exercises, progress in caring for the stump or prosthesis, and psychological reaction to the amputation.

7

GASTROINTESTINAL CARE

Disorders of the GI tract affect nearly everyone at some time. These conditions, which are tied to psychological health and stability, range from simple changes in bowel habits to life-threatening disorders requiring major surgery. Some GI conditions necessitate radical lifestyle or body image changes.

Nursing care focuses on treating the signs and symptoms, which vary widely among GI conditions and among patients. It also focuses on encouraging the patient to perform self-care and providing the patient support so he can adapt to the changes the condition or cure creates in his life.

Abdominal paracentesis assistance

Abdominal paracentesis is a bedside procedure that involves aspiration of fluid from the peritoneal space through a needle, trocar, or cannula inserted in the abdominal wall. It's used to diagnose and treat massive ascites resistant to other therapy. It helps determine the cause of ascites while relieving pressure created by ascites. It's used to detect intra-abdominal bleeding after traumatic injury and to obtain a peritoneal fluid specimen for laboratory analysis. It may precede other procedures, including radiography, peritoneal dialysis, and surgery. Nursing responsibilities include preparing the patient, monitoring the patient's condition, providing emotional support during the procedure, assisting the physician, and obtaining specimens for laboratory analysis.

CONTRAINDICATIONS
■ Use caution in pregnant patients, patients with bleeding tendencies, and patients with unstable vital signs.

EQUIPMENT

Tape measure ● sterile gloves ● clean gloves ● gown ● goggles ● linen-saver pads ● Vacutainer laboratory tubes ● large glass ● Vacutainer bottles (1,000 ml or larger) ● dry, sterile pressure dressing ● laboratory request forms ● povidone-iodine solution ● local anesthetic (multidose vial of 1% or 2% lidocaine with epinephrine) ● 4″ × 4″ sterile gauze pads ● paracentesis tray (containing needle, trocar, cannula, three-way stopcock), usually disposable ● sterile drapes ● marking pen ● 5-ml syringe with 22G or 25G needle ● alcohol pad ● 50-ml syringe ● suture materials ● salt-poor or 5% albumin ● povidone-iodine ointment (optional)

PREPARATION OF EQUIPMENT

▪ Check the sterility and expiration of the prepackaged tray.
▪ Assemble all equipment at the patient's bedside.

ESSENTIAL STEPS

▪ Wear clean gloves, a gown, and goggles.
▪ Verify the patient's identity using two patient identifiers, such as the patient's name and identification number.
▪ Reinforce the explanation of the procedure to the patient.
▪ Remind the patient that he shouldn't feel pain but may feel a stinging sensation and pressure.
▪ Make sure signed consent was obtained.
▪ Have the patient void before the procedure.
▪ If the patient can't void, insert an indwelling urinary catheter, if ordered.
▪ Obtain and record baseline values, including vital signs, weight, and abdominal girth. Indicate the abdominal area measured with a felt-tipped marking pen. Baseline data will be used to monitor the patient's status.
▪ Help the patient sit up in bed, on the side of the bed, or in a chair so fluid accumulates in the lower abdomen.
▪ Expose the patient's abdomen from the diaphragm to the pubis.
▪ The team should take a "time out" to make sure that the right procedure is being done on the right patient at the right site.
▪ Keep the rest of the patient covered to avoid chills.
▪ Place a linen-saver pad under the patient.
▪ Remind the patient to stay as still as possible during the procedure.
▪ Wash your hands.
▪ Open the paracentesis tray using sterile technique.
▪ Place the patient in a supine position, if ordered.

- The physician will prepare the patient's abdomen with povidone-iodine solution, cover the operative site with sterile drapes, and give the local anesthetic.
- If the paracentesis tray doesn't contain a sterile ampule of anesthetic, wipe the top of a multidose vial of anesthetic solution with an alcohol pad and invert the vial at a 45-degree angle to allow the physician to insert the sterile 5-ml syringe with the 22G or 25G needle and withdraw the anesthetic without touching the nonsterile vial.
- The physician may make a small incision before he inserts the needle or trocar and cannula (usually 1″ to 2″ [2.5 to 5 cm] below the umbilicus).
- The physician will listen for a popping sound. This signifies that the needle or trocar has pierced the peritoneum.
- Help the physician collect specimens (usually a cell count and culture) in proper containers.
- If the physician orders substantial drainage, connect the three-way stopcock and tubing to the cannula.
- Run the other end of the tubing to a large sterile Vacutainer or to a bag to allow gravity drainage; or aspirate the fluid with a three-way stopcock and 60-ml syringe.
- Gently turn the patient from side to side to enhance drainage.
- As the fluid drains, monitor the patient's vital signs every 15 minutes.
- Monitor the patient closely for vertigo, faintness, diaphoresis, pallor, heightened anxiety, tachycardia, dyspnea, and hypotension—especially if more than 1,500 ml of peritoneal fluid is aspirated at one time, which may induce a fluid shift and hypovolemic shock. Immediately report signs of shock to the physician.
- The physician may order the tube to be temporarily clamped after a certain amount is drained (usually over 1,500 ml).
- A salt-poor albumin or normal saline bolus may be ordered I.V. to prevent hypovolemia and a decline in renal function.
- Depending on the amount of drainage, a dressing or an ostomy bag may be applied over the puncture site to allow for the site to drain after the needle or trocar and cannula are removed.
- Wearing sterile gloves, apply the povidone-iodine ointment and dry, sterile pressure dressing to the site.
- Help the patient into a comfortable position.
- Monitor the patient's vital signs and the dressing for drainage every 15 minutes for 1 hour, every 30 minutes for 2 hours, every hour for 4 hours, and then every 4 hours for 24 hours to detect delayed reactions to the procedure.

- Note the color, amount, and character of drainage.
- Label the specimen tubes and send them to the laboratory with request forms.
- If the patient is receiving antibiotics, note this on the request form.
- Remove and dispose of all equipment properly.

SPECIAL CONSIDERATIONS

- If the patient has had paracentesis in the past, he may have scar tissue in the peritoneum, which creates smaller pockets of ascites. A preprocedure ultrasound may be performed to mark the pockets and make it easier for the physician to drain them.
- Help the patient remain still throughout the procedure.
- If the patient shows signs of hypovolemic shock, reduce the vertical distance between the needle or the trocar and cannula and the drainage collection container to slow the drainage rate. If necessary, temporarily clamp the tubing to stop the drainage.
- To prevent fluid shifts and hypovolemia, limit aspirated fluid to between 1,500 and 2,000 ml, or drain as ordered.
- If peritoneal fluid doesn't flow easily, reposition the patient, ensure all tubing clamps are open, and ensure there isn't any peritoneal tissue clogging the tubing.
- Verify suction in the Vacutainer collection bottle when you connect it to the drainage tubing.
- Use macrodrip tubing without a backflow device. The chamber or the spike end of the tubing can become clogged with peritoneal tissue. Monitor the tubing closely and change it, if necessary.
- After the procedure, observe for peritoneal fluid leakage and notify the physician if this develops.
- Maintain daily patient weight and abdominal girth records and compare these values with the baseline figures.
- Reinforce the explanation of the procedure to the patient.
- Remind the patient that he need not restrict fluids and food but that he may need to restrict sodium intake to prevent the reaccumulation of ascites.
- Provide support to decrease the patient's anxiety during the procedure.
- Reinforce with the patient that ascites may accumulate.

COMPLICATIONS

Complications include hypotension, oliguria, hyponatremia, perforation of abdominal organs, wound infection, peritonitis, and shock.

If more than 2 L of fluid is removed, ascitic fluid tends to form again.

DOCUMENTATION
■ Record the date and time of procedure.
■ Note the puncture site location.
■ Document how the wound was cleaned and dressed after the procedure.
■ Record the amount, color, viscosity, and odor of ascites drainage in your notes and on the fluid intake and output record.
■ Note the patient's vital signs, weight, and abdominal girth measurements before and after the procedure.
■ Document the patient's tolerance of the procedure.
■ Record signs and symptoms of complications during the procedure.
■ Note the number of specimens sent to the laboratory.
■ Record albumin or normal saline bolus administered on the intake and output record.

Continent ileostomy care

The continent, or pouch, ileostomy (also called a *Koch ileostomy* or an *ileal pouch*) has an internal reservoir fashioned from the terminal ileum. A continent ileostomy is an alternative to conventional ileostomy and may be used for a patient who requires proctocolectomy for chronic ulcerative colitis or multiple polyposis. Some patients may have a traditional ileostomy converted to a continent ileostomy.

CONTRAINDICATIONS
■ Crohn's disease
■ Morbid obesity
■ Patients requiring emergency surgery
■ Patients who are unable to care for the pouch

EQUIPMENT
Leg drainage bag ● bedside drainage bag ● normal saline solution ● 60-ml catheter-tip syringe ● extra continent ileostomy catheter ● 20-ml syringe with adapter ● 4″ × 4″ × 1″ foam dressing and Montgomery straps ● precut drain dressing ● gloves ● water-soluble lubricant ● graduated container ● skin sealant ● commercial catheter securing device (optional)

ESSENTIAL STEPS

■ The length of preoperative hospitalization varies with the patient's condition.

■ Preoperative nursing responsibilities include providing cleaning of the bowel with bowel preparation, antibiotic therapy, and emotional support.

■ After surgery, nursing responsibilities include ensuring patency of the drainage catheter, monitoring GI function and the condition of the stoma, performing peristomal and perineal skin care, and managing pain.

■ Daily reinforcement of teaching on pouch intubation and drainage begins as soon as possible after surgery.

■ Continuous drainage is maintained for 2 to 6 weeks to allow suture lines to heal.

■ During healing, a drainage catheter is attached to provide intermittent suction.

■ After the suture line heals, the patient learns to drain the pouch himself.

■ Nursing interventions for a patient undergoing surgery to create a continent ileostomy include standard preoperative and postoperative care, pouch care, and reinforcing patient teaching.

Preoperative care

■ Reinforce and supplement the physician's explanation of the procedure and implications for the patient.

■ Determine patient and family attitudes about the operation and forthcoming changes to the patient's body.

■ Provide encouragement and emotional support.

■ Verify the patient's identify using two patient identifiers, such as the patient's name and identification number.

■ Make sure that an informed consent form has been signed.

■ Make sure the operative site has been marked and all relevant documentation is complete.

■ Review orders for and administer bowel preparation, monitor antibiotic and I.V. fluid infusions, make sure the patient doesn't eat or drink after midnight the night before surgery, and ensure on-call medications are administered.

■ Make sure the patient has easy access to a bathroom or a commode during and after administration of the bowel preparation.

■ Monitor the patient for signs of dehydration during and after bowel preparation administration.

■ Monitor the patient's stools to ensure that they're clear, if ordered, before surgery.

Postoperative care

■ When the patient returns to his room, attach the drainage catheter emerging from the ileostomy to continuous gravity drainage.

■ A leg drainage bag may be attached to his thigh during ambulation.

■ Irrigate the catheter with 30 ml of normal saline solution, as ordered, to prevent obstruction and allow fluid return by gravity.

■ Immediately after surgery the drainage will be serosanguineous.

■ Monitor intake and output.

■ Check the catheter frequently when the patient begins eating solid food to ensure mucus and undigested food don't block it.

■ If the patient complains of abdominal cramps, distention, and nausea—symptoms of bowel obstruction—the catheter may be clogged.

■ Gently irrigate with 20 to 30 ml of water or normal saline solution until the catheter drains freely.

■ Move the catheter slightly or rotate gently to help clear the obstruction.

■ Try milking the catheter to clear the obstruction; notify the physician if this fails.

■ Check the stoma's size and observe for color, edema, bleeding, and viability every 2 hours for the first 24 hours, then every 4 hours for 48 to 72 hours.

RED FLAG *Normally pink to red or bright red and slightly edematous in the immediate postoperative period, a stoma that turns dark red, blue-red, pale, or cyanotic or blanches when touched may be ischemic.*

■ To care for the stoma and peristomal skin, put on gloves.

■ Remove the dressing, gently clean peristomal area with water, and pat dry.

■ Use skin sealant around the stoma to prevent skin irritation.

■ A stoma dressing can be applied by slipping a precut drain dressing around the catheter.

■ Cut a hole slightly larger than the lumen of the catheter in the center of a 4″ × 4″ × 1″ piece of foam.

■ Disconnect the catheter from the drainage bag and insert the distal end of the catheter through the hole in the foam and slide it onto the dressing.

■ Secure it with Montgomery straps.

■ Secure the catheter by wrapping the strap ties around it or use a commercial catheter-securing device.

■ Reconnect the catheter to the drainage bag.

■ The drainage catheter will be removed by the surgeon when he determines that the suture line has healed.
■ Monitor the peristomal skin for irritation from moisture.
■ To reduce discomfort from gas, encourage early and frequent ambulation.
■ To minimize gas pains, reinforce that the patient should avoid swallowing air, chew food well, limit talking while eating, and not drink from a straw. He should also avoid drinking fluids while eating and avoid carbonated beverages.

Draining the pouch
■ Provide privacy, reinforce the explanation of the procedure, and wash your hands.
■ Put on gloves.
■ Have the patient sit on the toilet to make him more comfortable during the procedure.
■ Remove the stoma dressing.
■ Encourage the patient to relax his abdominal muscles by taking several deep breaths to allow the catheter to slide easily into the pouch.
■ Lubricate the tip of the drainage catheter with the water-soluble lubricant and insert it into the stoma.
■ Gently push the catheter downward.
■ Direction of insertion may vary by patient.
■ When the catheter reaches the nipple valve of the internal pouch or reservoir (after 2″ to 2½″ [5 to 6.5 cm]), you'll feel resistance.
■ Tell the patient to take a deep breath as you exert gentle pressure on the catheter to insert it through the valve.
■ If this fails, have the patient lie in a supine position and rest for a few minutes, then try again.
■ Advance the catheter to the suture marking made by the surgeon.
■ Let the pouch drain completely. It usually takes 5 to 10 minutes, but with thick drainage or a clogged catheter, may take 30 minutes.
■ If the tube clogs, irrigate it with 30 ml of water or normal saline solution using the 60-ml catheter-tip syringe.
■ Rotate and milk the tube.
■ If these steps fail, remove, rinse, and reinsert the catheter.
■ Remove the catheter after completing drainage.
■ Measure output, subtracting the amount of irrigant used.
■ Rinse the catheter thoroughly with warm water.
■ Clean the peristomal area and apply a fresh stoma dressing.

SPECIAL CONSIDERATIONS

- Never aspirate fluid from the catheter because resulting negative pressure may damage surrounding tissue.
- Encourage the patient to relax. The first few times you intubate, he may be tense, making insertion difficult.
- To shorten drainage time, have the patient cough, press gently on his abdomen over the pouch, or suddenly tighten and relax his abdominal muscles.
- Monitor intake and output to ensure fluid and electrolyte balance.
- Average daily output should be at least 1,000 ml.
- *RED FLAG Report inadequate or excessive output (more than 1,400 ml daily).*
- Reinforce teaching the patient how to properly intubate and drain pouch independently and monitor his progress.
- Provide the patient with appropriate equipment.
- If the postoperative drainage catheter is still in place, reinforce proper care.
- Make sure the patient has a pouch-draining schedule and the appropriate pamphlets or audiovisual instructions.
- Make sure that the patient feels comfortable calling the physician, nurse, or other caregivers to ask questions or discuss problems.
- Remind the patient where and how to obtain supplies.
- Refer the patient to a local ostomy group.
- Reinforce dietary counseling and refer the patient to the nutritionist.
- Provide support related to body image disturbances and refer for counseling, if necessary.

COMPLICATIONS

Complications include obstruction, fistula, pouch perforation, nipple valve dysfunction, abscesses, diarrhea, skin irritation, stenosis of the stoma, and bacterial overgrowth in the pouch.

DOCUMENTATION

- Describe preoperative and postoperative care.
- Document catheter flushes.
- Note the condition of the stoma and peristomal skin.
- Record the patient's diet, drugs administered, and intubations.
- Note reinforced patient teaching and the patient's response.
- Document discharge planning.
- Document output from the ileostomy or catheter.

Gastrostomy feeding button care

A gastrostomy feeding button is used as an alternative feeding device for an ambulatory patient receiving long-term enteral feedings. It's approved for 6-month implantation and can replace gastrostomy tubes. The button is inserted into an established stoma (takes less than 15 minutes) and lies almost flush with skin; only the top of the safety plug is visible. Advantages over ordinary feeding tubes include cosmetic appeal, ease of maintenance, reduced skin irritation and breakdown, and less chance of being dislodged or migrating. The button has a one-way antireflux valve inside a mushroom dome that prevents leakage of gastric contents; it's usually replaced every 3 to 4 months, typically because the antireflux valve wears out.

CONTRAINDICATIONS
■ Intestinal obstruction that prohibits use of the bowel
■ Diffuse peritonitis
■ Intractable vomiting
■ Paralytic ileus
■ Severe diarrhea that makes metabolic management difficult
■ Use cautiously in patients with severe pancreatitis, enterocutaneous fistulae, and GI ischemia

EQUIPMENT
Gastrostomy feeding button of correct size (or all three sizes, if correct one isn't known) ● obturator ● water-soluble lubricant ● gloves ● feeding accessories, including adapter, feeding catheter, food syringe or bag, and formula ● catheter clamp ● cleaning equipment, including water, a syringe, cotton-tipped applicator, pipe cleaner, and mild soap ● I.V. pole, pump to provide continuous infusion over several hours (optional)

ESSENTIAL STEPS
■ Reinforce the explanation of the insertion, reinsertion, and feeding procedure to the patient. (See *How to assist with a gastrostomy feeding button reinsertion,* page 184.)
■ Verify the patient's identity using two patient identifiers, such as the patient's name and identification number.
■ Make sure signed consent has been obtained.

Providing feedings through the feeding button
■ Wash your hands and put on gloves.

How to assist with a gastrostomy feeding button reinsertion

If a gastrostomy feeding button pops out, assist the physician to perform these procedures to reinsert the device.

PREPARE EQUIPMENT
● Collect the feeding button (as shown); wash it with soap and water; rinse thoroughly and dry. Also obtain an obturator and water-soluble lubricant.

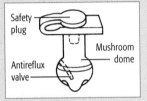

Safety plug

Mushroom dome

Antireflux valve

INSERT THE BUTTON
● Check the depth of the patient's stoma to make sure you have a feeding button of the correct size; clean around the stoma.
● Lubricate the obturator with water-soluble lubricant and distend the button several times to ensure the patency of the antireflux valve within the button.
● Lubricate the mushroom dome and stoma. Push the button through the stoma into the stomach (as shown).

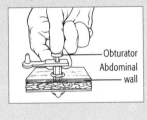

Obturator
Abdominal wall

● Remove the obturator by rotating it as you withdraw it to keep the antireflux valve from adhering to it. If the valve sticks, push the obturator back into the button until the valve closes.
● After removing the obturator, make sure the valve is closed.
● Close the flexible safety plug, which should be relatively flush with the skin surface (as shown).

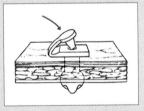

● If you need to give a feeding right away, open the safety plug and attach the feeding adapter and feeding tube (as shown). Deliver feeding as ordered.

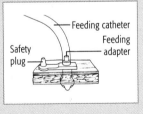

Feeding catheter

Feeding adapter

Safety plug

- Monitor the patient's bowel sounds. If absent, withhold the feeding and notify the physician.
- Attach the adapter and feeding catheter to the syringe or feeding bag.
- Clamp the catheter and fill the syringe or bag and catheter with formula.
- Open the safety plug and attach the adapter and feeding catheter to the button.
- Elevate the syringe or feeding bag above stomach level, and gravity-feed the formula for 15 to 30 minutes, varying the height as needed to alter infusion rate.
- Use an administration pump for a continuous infusion or for feedings lasting several hours.
- Refill the syringe before it's empty to prevent air from entering the stomach and distending the abdomen.
- After the feeding, flush the button with 10 ml of water.
- Lower the syringe or bag below stomach level to allow burping.
- Remove the adapter and feeding catheter; the antireflux valve should prevent gastric reflux.
- Snap the safety plug in place to keep the lumen clean and prevent leakage if the antireflux valve fails.
- If the patient feels nauseated or vomits after the feeding, vent the button with the adapter and feeding catheter to control emesis.
- Wash the catheter and syringe or feeding bag in warm, soapy water and rinse thoroughly.
- Clean the catheter and adapter with a pipe cleaner.
- Rinse well before using for the next feeding.
- Soak the equipment weekly, or according to manufacturer's recommendations.

SPECIAL CONSIDERATIONS

- Keep an extra feeding button at the bedside. If the button pops out during the feeding, notify the physician, help him to reinsert it, estimate the formula already delivered, and resume the feeding.
- Once daily, clean the peristomal skin with mild soap and water or povidone-iodine. Let the skin air-dry for 20 minutes to avoid skin irritation.
- Clean the peristomal site whenever the feeding bag is spilled.
- Reinforce with the patient how the gastrostomy feeding button is inserted and cared for.
- Remind the patient how to use the button for feedings.

◼ Reinforce how to clean the equipment and provide peristomal skin care.
◼ Tell the patient whom to call with questions.

COMPLICATIONS

Complications include nausea and vomiting, abdominal distention, exit-site infection, exit-site leakage, and peritonitis.

DOCUMENTATION

◼ Note the date, time, and duration of the feeding.
◼ Record the amount and type of feeding formula used.
◼ Document the patient's tolerance of the procedure.
◼ Note intake and output.
◼ Record the appearance of the stoma and surrounding skin.
◼ Document skin care.
◼ Document the presence of bowel sounds and a description of the patient's GI status.

Nasoenteric-decompression tube care

A nasoenteric-decompression tube is inserted by a physician or nurse practitioner nasally and advanced beyond the stomach into the intestinal tract. The patient requires encouragement and support while the tube is in place. Care involves continuous monitoring to ensure tube patency, proper suction, and bowel decompression and to detect complications, such as skin breakdown and fluid-electrolyte imbalances.

CONTRAINDICATIONS

◼ Nasal polyps, deviated septum, or other obstruction that prevents insertion.

EQUIPMENT

Suction apparatus with continuous or intermittent suction capability, depending on the physician's order (stationary or portable unit) ◼ container of water ◼ intake and output record sheets ◼ mouthwash and water mixture ◼ sponge-tipped swabs ◼ water-soluble lubricant ◼ cotton-tipped applicators ◼ safety pin ◼ tape or rubber band ◼ disposable irrigation set ◼ irrigant ◼ labels for tube lumens ◼ throat comfort measures such as gargle, viscous lidocaine, throat lozenges, ice collar, sour hard candy, or gum (optional)

PREPARATION OF EQUIPMENT

■ Assemble the suction apparatus and set up the suction unit.

■ Test the unit to make sure that the suction works.

ESSENTIAL STEPS

■ Verify the patient's identity using two patient identifiers, such as the patient's name and identification number.

■ Reinforce the explanation of the procedure to the patient and family and answer questions.

■ After tube insertion, have the patient lie on his right side for about 2 hours to promote the tube's passage.

■ After the tube advances past the pylorus, the physician or nurse practitioner can advance it 2″ (5 cm) per hour.

■ After it advances to the desired position, coil excess external tubing and secure it to the patient's gown or bed linens; secure the tube's position by taping it to the patient's face.

■ Maintain slack in the tubing so the patient can move safely in bed and so it doesn't cause pressure on the nares.

■ Remind the patient to call for assistance when getting out of bed.

■ After securing the tube, connect it to the tubing on the suction machine to begin decompression.

■ Check the suction machine every 2 hours to confirm proper function, tube patency, and bowel decompression.

■ Excessive negative pressure may draw the mucosa into the tube openings, impair the suction's effectiveness, and injure the mucosa. Intermittent suction may prevent these problems.

■ To check the functioning in an intermittent suction unit, look for drainage in the connecting tube and dripping into the collecting container.

■ Empty the drainage container or mark the drainage level with the time and date every 8 hours. Record output.

■ After decompression and before extubation, as ordered, provide a clear-to-full liquid diet and monitor bowel function.

■ Record intake and output to monitor fluid balance.

■ If you irrigate the tube, its length may prohibit aspiration of the irrigant; so record the amount of instilled irrigant as "intake."

■ Normal saline solution is preferred over water as an irrigant.

■ Monitor the patient for signs and symptoms of pneumonia since he may be unable to clear his pharynx or cough effectively with a tube in place.

■ Be alert for fever, chest pain, tachypnea or labored breathing, and diminished breath sounds over the affected area.

- Observe the characteristics of the drainage, including color, amount, consistency, odor, and unusual changes.
- Provide mouth care frequently and encourage the patient to brush his teeth or rinse his mouth with the mouthwash and water mixture.
- Lubricate the patient's lips with petroleum jelly using a cotton-tipped applicator.
- At least every 4 hours, clean and lubricate his external nostrils with water-soluble lubricant on a cotton-tipped applicator to prevent skin breakdown.
- Monitor the patient for peristalsis, signaled by bowel sounds, passage of flatus, decreased abdominal distention and, possibly, a spontaneous bowel movement, before resuming.

SPECIAL CONSIDERATIONS

- For a Miller-Abbott tube, clamp the lumen leading to the mercury balloon and label it "Do Not Touch."

    RED FLAG Observe the patient with a Miller-Abbott tube for signs of mercury toxicity, which can occur if the balloon ruptures. Signs and symptoms include nausea, diarrhea, vision disturbances, and dyspnea.

- Label the other lumen "Suction." Marking the tube may help prevent the accidental instillation of irrigant into the wrong lumen.
- If the suction machine doesn't work, replace it immediately.
- If the machine works properly but no drainage accumulates in the collection container, there may be an obstruction in the tube.
- As ordered, irrigate the tube with the irrigation set to clear the obstruction. (See *Clearing a nasoenteric-decompression tube obstruction*.)
- If the tube connects to a portable suction unit, the patient may move short distances while connected to the unit.
- If ordered, the tube can be disconnected briefly and clamped while the patient moves about.
- For throat irritation, offer mouthwash, gargles, viscous lidocaine, throat lozenges, an ice collar, sour hard candy, or gum, as ordered.
- If the tip of the balloon falls below the ileocecal valve (confirmed by X-ray), the tube can't be removed nasally. It must be advanced and removed through the anus.

    RED FLAG If the balloon at the end of the tube protrudes from the anus, notify the physician immediately.

- Reinforce the explanation of the purpose of the procedure and advise the patient about what to expect during and after insertion.

EQUIPMENT CHALLENGE

Clearing a nasoenteric-decompression tube obstruction

If the tube appears to be obstructed, notify the physician right away. He may order the following measures to restore patency:

● Disconnect the tube from the suction source and irrigate with normal saline solution. Use gravity flow to help clear the obstruction unless ordered otherwise.

● If irrigation doesn't reestablish patency, the tube may be obstructed by its position against the gastric mucosa. Tug slightly on the tube to move it away from the mucosa.

● If gentle tugging doesn't restore patency, the tube may be kinked and may need additional manipulation. Before proceeding, use the following guidelines:

– If the patient has had GI surgery, don't reposition or irrigate a nasoenteric-decompression tube without a physician's order.

– Avoid manipulating a tube that was inserted during surgery to avoid disturbing new sutures.

– Don't try to reposition a tube in a patient who was difficult to intubate.

■ Remind the patient of the signs and symptoms to report.
■ Keep the patient updated about the physician's approximation of when the tube will be removed.

COMPLICATIONS
Complications include fluid and electrolyte imbalance, pneumonia, mercury poisoning (from a ruptured mercury-filled balloon), and intussusception of the bowel.

DOCUMENTATION
■ Record the frequency and type of mouth and nose care given.
■ Note the therapeutic effect.
■ Document the amount, color, consistency, and odor of drainage.
■ Record the amount of drainage on intake and output sheet.
■ Note the amount of any irrigant or other fluid introduced through the tube or taken orally by the patient.
■ Document the amount of suction applied to the tube.
■ Note the amount and character of vomitus.
■ Record the patient's tolerance of the insertion and removal.
■ Document a description of the patient's GI status including the presence of bowel sounds, whether or not the patient reports flatus, and any bowel movements.

Nasogastric tube care

A nasogastric tube is inserted through the nose and is passed into the stomach. It can be used for decompression, lavage, gastric emptying, and occasionally short-term feedings. After a nasogastric (NG) tube is inserted, careful monitoring of the patient and equipment is required. Specific care varies only slightly for the most commonly used NG tubes (the single-lumen Levin tube and the double-lumen Salem sump tube).

CONTRAINDICATIONS
None known.

EQUIPMENT
Irrigant (usually normal saline solution) ● irrigant container ● 60-ml catheter-tip syringe ● bulb syringe ● suction equipment ● sponge-tipped swabs or toothbrush and toothpaste ● petroleum jelly ● ½" or 1" hypoallergenic tape ● water-soluble lubricant ● gloves ● pH test strip ● linen-saver pad ● emesis basin (optional)

PREPARATION OF EQUIPMENT
■ Make sure the suction equipment works properly. (See *Common gastric suction devices.*)
■ When using a Salem sump tube with suction, connect the larger, primary lumen (for drainage and suction) to the suction equipment and select the appropriate setting, as ordered (usually low continuous suction).
■ A Levin tube usually calls for intermittent low suction.

ESSENTIAL STEPS
■ Verify the patient's identity using two patient identifiers, such as the patient's name and identification number.
■ Reinforce the explanation of the procedure to the patient and provide privacy.
■ Wash your hands and put on gloves.

Irrigating a nasogastric tube
■ Review the irrigation schedule (usually every 4 hours).
  RED FLAG Check the physician's orders before irrigating an NG tube. Postoperative patients, such as those who have undergone an esophagogastrectomy, a partial gastrectomy, or a Whipple procedure, may have "Do Not Move, Do Not Irrigate" orders.

Common gastric suction devices

Various suction devices are available for applying negative pressure to nasogastric (NG) and other drainage tubes. Two common types are shown here.

PORTABLE SUCTION MACHINE

In the portable suction machine, a vacuum created by an electric pump draws gastric contents up the NG tube and into the collecting bottle.

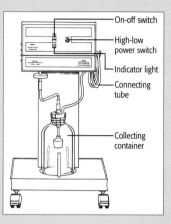

- On-off switch
- High-low power switch
- Indicator light
- Connecting tube
- Collecting container

STATIONARY SUCTION MACHINE

A stationary wall-unit apparatus can provide intermittent or continuous suction. On-off switches and variable power settings let you set and adjust the suction force on either machine.

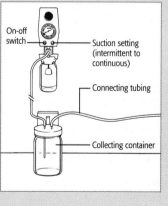

- On-off switch
- Suction setting (intermittent to continuous)
- Connecting tubing
- Collecting container

■ Aspirate stomach contents to check correct positioning in the stomach and prevent the patient from aspirating the irrigant.

◼ Examine the aspirate and place a small amount on the pH test strip. Correct gastric placement is likely if the aspirate has a gastric fluid appearance (grassy-green, clear and colorless with mucus shreds, or brown) and the pH, if bedside testing is allowed at the facility, is 5.0 or less. If bedside or waived testing isn't allowed, a specimen can be sent to the laboratory for a pH reading.

◼ Measure the amount of irrigant (usually 10 to 30 ml) in a syringe (bulb or 60-ml catheter-tip) for accurate input and output monitoring.

◼ When using suction with a Salem sump tube or a Levin tube, unclamp and disconnect the tube from the suction equipment while holding it over a linen-saver pad or an emesis basin.

◼ Slowly instill the irrigant into the NG tube.

◼ Aspirate the solution with the bulb syringe or a 60-ml catheter-tip syringe. All of the irrigant should be returned. If not, the tube may need to be repositioned.

◼ Report any bleeding.

◼ Reconnect the tube to suction after completing irrigation.

Instilling a solution through a nasogastric tube

◼ If the physician orders instillation, inject the solution and don't aspirate it.

◼ Note the amount of instilled solution on the intake and output record.

◼ Check the physician's orders to determine whether he wants suction to be held for a time while the instilled solution is absorbed. Reattach the tube to suction as ordered.

◼ After attaching the Salem sump tube's primary lumen to suction, instill 10 to 20 cc of air into the vent lumen to verify patency.

◼ Listen for a soft hiss in the vent. If you don't hear this sound, the tube may be clogged.

◼ Recheck patency by instilling 10 ml of normal saline solution and 10 to 20 cc of air in the vent.

Monitoring patient comfort and condition

◼ Provide mouth care once per shift or as needed.

◼ Depending on the patient's condition, use sponge-tipped swabs to clean his teeth or assist him with brushing.

◼ Coat the patient's lips with petroleum jelly.

◼ Every 4 to 8 hours, check the tape securing the tube to his nose, and change it as needed or at least daily. Clean the skin, apply a liquid skin barrier (if desired), apply fresh tape, and dab water-soluble lubricant on the nostrils as needed.

◼ Monitor GI status regularly.

- Measure the drainage from the tube and update intake and output record every 8 hours or as ordered.
- Monitor for electrolyte imbalances with excessive gastric output.
- Monitor the gastric drainage and note its color, consistency, and odor.
- Immediately report drainage that looks like coffee grounds or bright red blood.
- If you suspect the drainage contains blood, send a specimen for an occult blood screening or guaiac to the laboratory.

SPECIAL CONSIDERATIONS

- Irrigate the NG tube with 30 ml of irrigant before instilling a drug and instill 30 to 50 ml of water after the drug is administered to flush the tubing.

   LIFE STAGES For a child, instill only 15 to 30 ml of water after drug administration.

  RED FLAG When possible, use liquid forms of drugs. If they aren't available, crush pills well. Don't crush enteric-coated or sustained-released drugs, which lose their effectiveness when crushed.

- Wait about 30 minutes, or as ordered, after instillation before re-connecting suction equipment to allow sufficient time for the drug to be absorbed.
- When no drainage appears, check the suction equipment for proper function.
- Holding the NG tube over a linen-saver pad or emesis basin, separate the tube and the suction source.
- Check suction by placing the suction tubing in an irrigant container. If the apparatus draws water, check the NG tube for proper function.
- Note the amount of water drawn into the suction container on the intake and output record so that it's subtracted from the actual output of the tube.
- A dysfunctional NG tube may be clogged or incorrectly positioned. Attempt to irrigate the tube, reposition the patient, or rotate and reposition the tube. If the tube was inserted during surgery, if the patient is known to have esophageal varices, or if the physician has entered "do not move, do not irrigate" orders, avoid this maneuver to avoid interfering with gastric or esophageal sutures; notify the physician.
- If you can move the patient and interrupt suction, disconnect the NG tube from the suction equipment.
- Clamp the tube to prevent stomach contents from draining out of the tube.

- If the patient has a Salem sump tube, watch for gastric reflux in the vent lumen when pressure in the stomach exceeds atmospheric pressure.
- Monitor the suction equipment for proper functioning.
- Irrigate the NG tube and instill 30 cc of air into the vent tube to maintain patency. Don't attempt to stop reflux by clamping the vent tube.
- Unless contraindicated, elevate the patient's torso more than 30 degrees, and keep the vent tube above his midline to prevent a siphoning effect.
- Reinforce with the patient a description of the procedure and why it's being performed, as needed.
- Reinforce that the patient should ask for assistance getting out of bed so the tube doesn't move or dislodge.
- Remind the patient that he is not to have anything by mouth as long as the tube is in place, unless otherwise ordered by the physician.
- Provide viscous lidocaine or lidocaine spray to the back of the patient's throat if pain or irritation occurs, as ordered.

COMPLICATIONS

Complications include epigastric pain and vomiting; perforation; dehydration and electrolyte imbalances; nasal skin breakdown and discomfort; increased mucus secretions; aspiration pneumonia; damage of the gastric mucosa from suctioning; aggravation of esophagitis, ulcers, or esophageal varices causing hemorrhage; and pain, swelling, and salivary dysfunction, which may signal parotitis in dehydrated, debilitated patients.

DOCUMENTATION

- Note the aspiration of gastric contents and the pH of the drainage to confirm proper placement of the tube.
- Record fluid intake and output, including the instilled irrigant.
- Document the irrigation schedule, the actual time of each irrigation, and the amount used to irrigate and the amount returned.
- Note the color, consistency, odor, and amount of drainage.
- Record the times the tape was changed and the condition of the nostrils.
- Record the pH of aspirate and occult blood test results.
- Record serum laboratory values.
- Note the amount of suction applied to the tube.
- Describe how the patient tolerated the procedure.

Nasogastric tube insertion and removal

A nasogastric (NG) tube is usually inserted to decompress the stomach. The tube can prevent vomiting after major surgery. It's also used to assess and treat upper GI bleeding, collect gastric contents for analysis, perform gastric lavage, aspirate gastric secretions, and administer drugs. Sometimes it's used short-term for feedings. It requires close observation of the patient and verification of proper placement. The tube must be inserted with care in pregnant patients, patients with known esophageal varices, and patients with an increased risk of complications. Most common tubes are the Levin tube (one lumen) and Salem sump tube (two lumens [air flows through the vent lumen to protect the gastric mucosa should the tube adhere to the stomach lining]).

CONTRAINDICATIONS
■ Facial or basilar skull fracture with cribriform plate injury
■ Hypothermia (insertion can cause myocardial irritability leading to ventricular fibrillation)

EQUIPMENT
For inserting a nasogastric tube
Tube (usually #12, #14, #16, or #18 French for a normal adult) ●
towel or linen-saver pad ● facial tissues ● emesis basin ● penlight ●
1″ or 2″ hypoallergenic tape ● gloves ● water-soluble lubricant ●
cup or glass of water with straw (if appropriate) ● pH test strip ●
tongue blade ● catheter-tip or bulb syringe or irrigation set ● safety
pin ● ordered suction equipment

For removing a nasogastric tube
Stethoscope ● gloves ● catheter-tip syringe ● normal saline solution
● towel or linen-saver pad ● adhesive remover ● clamp (optional)

PREPARATION OF EQUIPMENT
■ Inspect the NG tube for defects.
■ Check the tube's patency by flushing it with water.

ESSENTIAL STEPS
■ Provide privacy.
■ Verify the patient's identity using two patient identifiers, such as the patient's name and identification number.
■ Wash your hands and put on gloves.

Inserting a nasogastric tube

- Reinforce the explanation of the procedure to the patient.
- Reinforce that swallowing will ease the tube's advancement down the esophagus and into the stomach. Coughing or gagging may cause the tube to advance down the trachea.
- Establish a signal that the patient can use if he wants you to stop briefly and rest during the procedure.
- Place the patient in high Fowler's position, unless contraindicated.
- Drape a towel or linen-saver pad over the patient's chest.
- Have the patient blow his nose to clear his nostrils.
- Place facial tissues and an emesis basin within the patient's reach.
- Help the patient face forward with his neck in a neutral position.
- To determine approximately how long the NG tube must be to reach the stomach, hold the end of the tube at the tip of the patient's nose, then extend the tube to his earlobe and down to the xiphoid process.
- Mark this distance on the tubing with tape. It may be necessary to add 2″ (5 cm) for tall individuals to ensure entry into the stomach.
- To determine which nostril will allow easier access, use a penlight and inspect for a deviated septum or other abnormalities, ask the patient if he ever had nasal surgery or a nasal injury, and monitor airflow in both nostrils.
- Lubricate the first 3″ (7.6 cm) of the tube with a water-soluble gel.
- Instruct the patient to hold his head straight and upright.
- Grasp the tube with the end pointing downward (curve it if necessary) and carefully insert it into the patient's more patent nostril.
- Aim the tube downward and toward the ear closer to the chosen nostril.
- Advance it slowly to avoid pressure on the turbinates and resultant pain and bleeding. When the tube reaches the nasopharynx, you'll feel resistance.
- Instruct the patient to slightly lower his chin to his chest to close the trachea and open the esophagus.
- Rotate the tube 180 degrees toward the opposite nostril.
- Unless contraindicated, offer the patient a cup or glass of water with a straw.
- Direct the patient to sip and swallow as you slowly advance the tube.
- Watch for respiratory distress as you advance the tube.
- Stop advancing the tube when the tape mark reaches the patient's nostril.
- Secure the tube to the patient's nostril with a piece of tape.

BEST PRACTICE

Confirming nasogastric tube placement

Confirming nasogastric (NG) tube placement after insertion and while it's in place helps prevent complications, such as perforation of the esophagus and pulmonary conditions (bleeding, aspiration, pneumonitis, empyema, pleural effusion, and pneumothorax).

● Use a tongue blade and penlight to examine the patient's mouth and throat for signs of a coiled section of tubing.

● Attach a catheter-tip or bulb syringe and try to aspirate stomach contents.

● Examine the aspirate and place a small amount on the pH test strip.

● Correct gastric placement is likely if the aspirate has a typical gastric fluid appearance (grassy-green, clear and colorless with mucus shreds, or brown) and pH is 5.0 or less.

● If you still can't aspirate stomach contents, position the patient on his left side to move the contents into the greater curvature of the stomach and aspirate again.

● If that doesn't yield gastric contents, inject 10 cc of air into the tube; then advance or pull the tube back 1" to 2" (2.5 to 5 cm). Then try to aspirate stomach contents.

● If tests don't confirm proper tube placement, X-ray verification will be needed.

● Secure the NG tube to the patient's nose with hypoallergenic tape.

● Alternatively, stabilize the tube with a prepackaged product that secures and cushions it at the nose.

● Notify the physician and await an X-ray.

Ensuring proper tube placement

■ Once the tube is positioned, correct placement must be confirmed. (See *Confirming nasogastric tube placement.*)

RED FLAG When confirming tube placement, never place the tube's end in a container of water. If the tube is in the trachea, the patient may aspirate water. Bubbles don't confirm proper placement because the tube may be coiled in the trachea or the esophagus.

Fastening and connecting the tube

■ Tie a slipknot around the tube with a rubber band, then secure the rubber band to the patient's gown with a safety pin.

■ Fasten the tape tab to the patient's gown.

■ Attach the tube to suction equipment, if ordered, and set the designated suction pressure. Monitor for drainage.

■ Provide frequent nose and mouth care while the tube is in place.

Removing a nasogastric tube

- Reinforce the explanation of the procedure to the patient.
- Monitor bowel function by auscultating for peristalsis or flatus.
- Help the patient into semi-Fowler's position.
- Wash your hands and put on gloves.
- Drape a towel or linen-saver pad across the patient's chest.
- Using a catheter-tip syringe, flush the tube with 10 ml of normal saline solution to ensure that the tube doesn't contain stomach contents.
- Untape the tube from the patient's nose and unpin it from his gown.
- Clamp the tube by folding it in your hand.
- Ask the patient to hold his breath to close the epiglottis.
- Slowly withdraw the tube.
- Immediately cover and discard the tube.
- Assist the patient with thorough mouth and skin care.
- For the next 48 hours, monitor for signs of GI dysfunction and distention.
- GI dysfunction may necessitate reinsertion of the tube.

SPECIAL CONSIDERATIONS

- Unless otherwise ordered by the physician, the patient should take nothing by mouth while the tube is in place.
- If the tube position can't be confirmed, the physician may order fluoroscopy to verify placement.
- If the patient has a deviated septum or other nasal condition that prevents nasal insertion, pass the tube orally. Sliding the tube over the tongue, proceed as you would for nasal insertion.
- When using the oral route, coil the end of the tube around your hand.
- If the patient is unconscious, tilt his chin toward his chest to close the trachea.
- Advance the tube between respirations.
- While advancing the tube, watch for signs that it entered the trachea, such as choking or breathing difficulties in a conscious patient and cyanosis or a decreased oxygen saturation in an unconscious patient or a patient without a cough reflex. If these signs occur, remove the tube immediately.
- Allow the patient time to rest, then try to reinsert the tube.
- After tube placement, vomiting suggests tubal obstruction or incorrect position. Monitor immediately to determine the cause.
- Most tablets and pills can be given through the tube by crushing them and diluting as necessary; clamping the NG tube from suc-

Giving drugs through a nasogastric tube

Verify the patient's identity using two patient identifiers. Verify nasogastric (NG) tube placement. Holding the NG tube above the patient's nose, irrigate the NG tube with 30 ml of irrigant, then pour up to 30 ml of diluted drug into the syringe barrel. To prevent air from entering the patient's stomach, hold the tube at a slight angle and add more drug before the syringe empties. If necessary, raise the tube slightly higher to increase infusion rate.

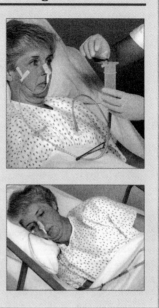

After you've delivered the entire dose, instill 30 to 50 ml of water to flush the tubing. Then clamp the NG tube and position the patient on her right side, head slightly elevated, to minimize esophageal reflux. Wait about 30 minutes, or as ordered, after administering the medication to reconnect the suction equipment.

tion for 20 to 30 minutes allows for absorption. (See *Giving drugs through a nasogastric tube*.)

▶ ***RED FLAG*** *Don't crush enteric-coated or sustained-released drugs, which lose their effectiveness when crushed. Drugs should be given in the liquid form if possible.*

- Check the physician's orders before administering drugs through an NG tube. If the patient doesn't exhibit any signs of bowel function, the physician may order the I.V. form of drugs when available so that there's no doubt about whether the drug was efficiently absorbed.
- Reinforce with the patient what to expect during insertion and what signs and symptoms to report.
- Reinforce that the patient should avoid food and drink for several hours after tube removal or as per the physician's orders.

COMPLICATIONS

Complications include skin erosion at the nostril, sinusitis, esophagitis, esophagotracheal fistula, gastric ulceration, pulmonary and oral infection, electrolyte imbalances, and dehydration.

DOCUMENTATION

- Record the type and size of the NG tube.
- Note the date, time, and route of insertion and removal.
- Note the patient's tolerance of procedure.
- Document the type, color, odor, consistency, and amount of gastric drainage.
- Record signs and symptoms of complications.
- Note irrigation procedures.
- Note GI findings following NG removal, such as nausea, vomiting, abdominal distention, food intolerance, and lack of bowel sounds or flatus.
- Document reinforced patient teaching and the patient's response.

Transabdominal tube feeding and care

To access the stomach, duodenum, or jejunum, the physician may place a tube through the patient's abdominal wall, either surgically or percutaneously. A gastrostomy or jejunostomy tube is usually inserted during intra-abdominal surgery. A gastrostomy tube may also be placed during a bedside endoscopy under moderate sedation. This procedure may be used for feeding during the immediate postoperative period or may provide long-term enteral access, depending on the type of surgery. Feedings may begin after 24 hours (or when peristalsis resumes). Eventually, a tube may need replacement; the physician may recommend a similar tube, such as an indwelling urinary catheter or a mushroom catheter, or a gastrostomy button.

CONTRAINDICATIONS

- Obstruction (such as esophageal stricture or duodenal blockage)
- Previous gastric surgery
- Morbid obesity
- Ascites

EQUIPMENT
For feeding

Feeding formula ● large-bulb or catheter-tip syringe ● 120 ml of water ● 4″ × 4″ gauze pads ● soap ● skin protectant ● hypoallergenic tape ● gravity-drip administration bags ● mouthwash, toothpaste, or mild saline solution ● stethoscope ● gloves ● enteral infusion pump (optional)

For decompression
Suction apparatus with tubing and straight drainage collection set

PREPARATION OF EQUIPMENT
■ Check the expiration date on commercially prepared feeding formulas.
■ If the formula has been prepared by the dietitian or pharmacist, check preparation time and date.
■ Discard opened formula more than 24 hours old.
■ Commercially prepared administration sets and enteral pumps allow continuous formula administration.
■ Place the desired amount of formula into the gavage container and purge air from the tubing.
■ To avoid contamination, hang only a 4- to 6-hour supply of formula at a time.

ESSENTIAL STEPS
■ Verify the patient's identity using two patient identifiers, such as the patient's name and identification number.
■ Provide privacy and wash your hands.
■ Reinforce the explanation of the procedure to the patient.
■ Monitor for bowel sounds and abdominal distention before feeding.
■ Ask the patient to sit or assist him into semi-Fowler's position.
■ For an intermittent feeding, have the patient maintain this position throughout the feeding and for 30 minutes to 1 hour afterward. For a continuous feeding, keep the head of the patient's bed elevated to at least 30 degrees to prevent aspiration.
■ Put on gloves.
■ Before starting the feeding, measure residual gastric contents.
■ Attach the syringe to the feeding tube and aspirate.

RED FLAG If contents measure more than twice the amount infused, or the amount determined by the physician, withhold the feeding and recheck in 1 hour. If residual contents remain too high, notify the physician; formula may not be absorbed properly. Residual contents are minimal with percutaneous endoscopic jejunostomy tube feedings.

■ Allow 30 ml of water to flow into the feeding tube to establish patency.
■ Be sure to give formula at room temperature.

Intermittent feedings

- Allow gravity to help the formula flow over 30 to 45 minutes.
- Begin intermittent feedings with a low volume (200 ml) daily. According to the patient's tolerance, increase volume per feeding, as needed, to reach the prescribed calorie intake.
- When the feeding is completed, flush the feeding tube with 30 to 60 ml of water. This maintains patency and provides hydration. Cap the tube to prevent leakage.
- Rinse the feeding administration set thoroughly with hot water to avoid contaminating subsequent feedings. Allow it to dry.

Continuous feedings

- Measure residual gastric contents before each feeding and every 4 hours.
- To administer the feeding with a pump, set up the equipment according to the manufacturer's guidelines and fill the feeding bag.
- To administer the feeding by gravity, fill the container with formula and purge air from the tubing before connecting it to the gastrostomy or jejunostomy tube.
- Monitor the gravity drip rate or pump infusion rate frequently to ensure accurate delivery.
- Flush the feeding tube with 30 to 60 ml of water before each feeding and every 4 hours to maintain patency and provide hydration.
- Monitor intake and output to detect fluid or electrolyte imbalances.

Decompression

- To decompress the stomach, connect the percutaneous endoscopic gastrostomy port to the suction device with tubing or straight gravity drainage tubing.

Tube exit site care

- Provide daily skin care.

  RED FLAG Always remove the dressing by hand. Never cut dressing away over the catheter since the catheter may be accidentally cut.

- At least daily and as needed, clean the skin around the tube's exit site using a 4" × 4" gauze pad soaked in prescribed cleaning solution and apply povidone-iodine ointment over the exit site. (See *Caring for a percutaneous endoscopic gastrostomy or jejunostomy site*.)

Caring for a percutaneous endoscopic gastrostomy or jejunostomy site

The exit site of a percutaneous endoscopic gastrostomy (PEG) or percutaneous endoscopic jejunostomy tube requires routine observation and care. Follow these care guidelines:

● Change the dressing daily while the tube is in place.

● After removing the dressing, carefully slide the tube's outer bumper away from the skin (as shown) about ½″ (1 cm).

● Monitor the skin around the tube and observe for redness and other signs of infection or erosion.

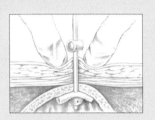

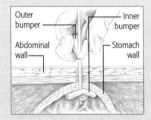

Outer bumper — Inner bumper
Abdominal wall — Stomach wall

● Gently depress the skin surrounding the tube and monitor for drainage (as shown above right). Expect minimal wound drainage initially after implantation. This should subside in about 1 week.

● Monitor the tube for wear and tear. (A tube that wears out will need replacement.)

● Clean the site with the prescribed cleaning solution. Apply povidone-iodine ointment over the exit site according to your facility's guidelines.

● Rotate the outer bumper 90 degrees (to avoid repeating the same tension on the same skin area) and slide the outer bumper back over the exit site.

● If leakage appears at the PEG site, or if the patient risks dislodging the tube, apply a sterile gauze dressing over the site. Don't put sterile gauze underneath the outer bumper. Loosening the anchor this way allows the feeding tube free play, which could lead to wound abscess.

● Write the date and time of the dressing change on the tape.

■ When healed, wash skin around the exit site daily with soap; rinse with water and dry.

■ Apply skin protectant, if necessary.

■ Anchor a gastrostomy or jejunostomy tube to the skin with hypoallergenic tape. Coil the tube, if necessary, and tape it to the abdomen.

SPECIAL CONSIDERATIONS

■ The physician may suture the tube in place to prevent leaking of gastric contents.

■ If the patient vomits or complains of nausea, feeling full, or regurgitation, stop the feeding immediately and monitor his condition.

■ Flush the feeding tube and attempt to restart the feeding again in 1 hour (measure residual gastric contents first). You may have to decrease the volume or rate of feedings.

🚩 *RED FLAG If the patient develops dumping syndrome (nausea, vomiting, cramps, pallor, diarrhea) the feedings may have been given too quickly.*

■ Brush all surfaces of the teeth, gums, and tongue at least twice daily using mouthwash, toothpaste, or mild saline solution.

■ You can give most tablets and pills through the tube by crushing them and diluting as necessary.

🚩 *RED FLAG Don't crush enteric-coated or sustained-released drugs, which lose their effectiveness when crushed. Use drugs in liquid form if possible.*

■ Control diarrhea resulting from dumping syndrome by using continuous pump or gravity-drip infusions, diluting the feeding formula, or adding antidiarrheal drugs.

🚩 *RED FLAG Send a stool specimen for culture before starting an antidiarrheal medication.*

■ If the tube falls out, cover the site and contact the physician.

■ Reinforce the instructions regarding all aspects of enteral feedings, including tube maintenance and site care, with the patient, family members, and other caregivers.

■ Reinforce the signs and symptoms to report to the physician, define emergency situations, and review actions to take.

COMPLICATIONS

Common complications related to transabdominal tubes include GI or other systemic problems; mechanical malfunction; metabolic disturbances; cramping, nausea, vomiting, bloating, and diarrhea; fat malabsorption; intestinal atrophy from malnutrition; and constipation from inadequate hydration or insufficient exercise. Systemic problems may be caused by pulmonary aspiration, infection at the tube exit site, and contaminated formula. Typical mechanical problems include tube dislodgment, obstruction, or tube migration; occlusion; and rupture or tube cracking from age, drying, or frequent manipulation. Monitor for vitamin and mineral deficiencies, glucose tolerance, and fluid and electrolyte imbalances, which may follow bouts of diarrhea or constipation.

DOCUMENTATION

■ On the intake and output record, note the date, time, amount of each feeding, and water volume instilled.

■ Maintain total volumes for nutrients and water separately to allow calculation of nutrient intake.

■ Document the type of formula, infusion method, and rate.

■ Record the patient's tolerance of procedure and formula.

■ Document the amount of residual gastric contents.

■ Record complications and a description of the patient's GI status.

■ Document reinforced patient teaching.

■ Note the patient's progress in self-care.

■ Document oral intake to determine the total calories ingested; keep a calorie count.

■ Record laboratory values including bedside blood glucose levels.

T-tube care

A T-tube (also called a *biliary draining tube*) may be placed in the common bile duct after cholecystectomy or choledochostomy. (See *Understanding T-tube placement,* page 206.)

The tube facilitates biliary drainage during healing. The surgeon inserts the short end (crossbar) into the common bile duct and draws the long end through an incision in the skin. The tube is then connected to a closed gravity drainage system. Postoperatively, it remains in place between 7 and 14 days.

CONTRAINDICATIONS
None known.

EQUIPMENT
Graduated collection container ● small plastic bag ● sterile gloves and clean gloves ● clamp ● sterile 4″ × 4″ gauze pads ● transparent dressings ● rubber band ● normal saline solution ● sterile cleaning solution ● two sterile basins ● povidone-iodine pads ● sterile precut drain dressings ● hypoallergenic paper tape ● skin protectant, such as petroleum jelly, aluminum-based gel, or zinc oxide ● Montgomery straps (optional)

PREPARATION OF EQUIPMENT
■ Assemble the equipment at the bedside.

■ Open all sterile equipment. Place one sterile 4″ × 4″ gauze pad in each sterile basin.

Understanding T-tube placement

The T tube is placed in the common bile duct, anchored to the abdominal wall, and connected to a closed drainage system.

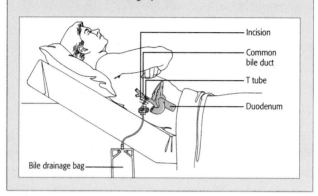

Incision

Common bile duct

T tube

Duodenum

Bile drainage bag

- Using sterile technique, pour 50 ml of cleaning solution into one basin and 50 ml of normal saline solution into the other basin.
- Tape a small plastic bag on the table to use for refuse.

ESSENTIAL STEPS

- Verify the patient's identity using two patient identifiers, such as the patient's name and identification number.
- Provide privacy and reinforce the explanation of the procedure to the patient.
- Wash your hands.

Emptying drainage

- Put on clean gloves.
- Place the graduated collection container under the outlet valve of the drainage bag. Without contaminating the clamp, valve, or outlet valve, empty the bag's contents completely into the container and reseal the outlet valve.
- Carefully measure and record the character, color, and amount of drainage.
- Discard the gloves.

Redressing the T-tube

- Wash your hands and put on clean gloves.

- Without dislodging the T-tube, remove old dressings, and dispose of them in the small plastic bag. Remove gloves.
- Wash your hands again and put on sterile gloves; follow strict sterile technique to prevent contamination of the incision.
- Monitor the incision and tube site for signs of infection, including erythema, edema, warmth, tenderness, induration, or skin excoriation. Monitor for wound dehiscence or evisceration.
- Use sterile cleaning solution as prescribed to clean the insertion site and remove dried matter or drainage from around the tube. Start at the tube site and gently wipe outward in a continuous motion to prevent recontamination of the incision.
- Use normal saline solution to rinse off the prescribed cleaning solution. Dry the area with a sterile 4″ × 4″ gauze pad and discard all used materials.
- Using a povidone-iodine pad, wipe the incision site in a circular motion. Allow the area to dry.
- Apply a skin protectant (petroleum jelly, zinc oxide, or aluminum-based gel) to prevent injury from draining bile.
- Apply a sterile precut drain dressing on each side of the T-tube to absorb drainage.
- Apply a sterile 4″ × 4″ gauze pad or transparent dressing over the T-tube and the drain dressings.

  ◤ **RED FLAG** *Don't kink the tubing, which can block drainage; and don't put the dressing over the open end of the T-tube because it connects to the closed drainage system.*

- Secure the dressings with the hypoallergenic paper tape or Montgomery straps if necessary.
- If the patient is ambulatory, pin or anchor the portable closed gravity drainage system to the patient so that if the bag becomes full and heavy, the weight doesn't dislodge the tube.

Clamping the T-tube
- As ordered, occlude the tube lightly with a clamp or wrap a rubber band around the end. Clamping the tube 1 hour before and after meals diverts bile back to the duodenum to aid digestion.
- Monitor the patient's response to clamping.
- To ensure his comfort and safety, check bile drainage amounts regularly.

  ◤ **RED FLAG** *Report signs of obstructed bile flow, such as chills, fever, tachycardia, nausea, right-upper-quadrant fullness and pain, jaundice, dark foamy urine, and clay-colored stools.*

SPECIAL CONSIDERATIONS
- The T-tube usually drains 300 to 500 ml of thin, blood-tinged bile in the first 24 hours after surgery.

RED FLAG *Report drainage that exceeds 500 ml in the first 24 hours after surgery. If it's 50 ml or less, notify the physician; the tube may be obstructed. Drainage typically declines to 200 ml or less after 4 days and the color changes to green-brown and it thickens. Monitor fluid, electrolyte, and acid-base status.*

■ To prevent excessive bile loss (over 500 ml in the first 24 hours) or backflow contamination, secure the T-tube drainage system at abdominal level. Bile will flow into the bag only when biliary pressure increases.
■ Provide meticulous skin care and frequent dressing changes since bile is irritating to the skin.
■ Monitor for bile leakage, which may indicate obstruction.
■ Monitor tube patency and the condition of the site hourly for the first 8 hours, then every 4 hours until the physician removes the tube.
■ Protect the skin edges and avoid excessive taping.
■ Monitor all urine and stools for color changes. Monitor for icteric skin and sclera and pruritus, which may signal jaundice.
■ Reinforce with the patient that loose bowels occur commonly the first few weeks after surgery.
■ Remind the patient about signs and symptoms of T-tube and biliary obstruction and to report them to the physician.
■ Teach the patient how to care for the tube at home.
■ Reinforce with the patient that bile stains clothing and is irritating to the skin.

COMPLICATIONS
Complications include obstructed bile flow, skin excoriation or breakdown, tube dislodgment, drainage reflux, and infection.

DOCUMENTATION
■ Record the date and time of each dressing change.
■ Write down the color, character, and volume of bile collected.
■ Record the color of skin and mucous membranes around the T tube.
■ Keep a precise record of temperature trends and the amount and frequency of urination and bowel movements.
■ Record reinforced patient teaching and the patient's response.

Tube feedings

Tube feedings deliver a liquid formula directly to the stomach (known as *gastric gavage*), duodenum, or jejunum. They're used for patients who can't eat normally because of dysphagia or oral or esophageal obstruction or injury. They may be given to an unconscious or intubated patient, to a patient recovering from GI tract surgery who can't eat food by mouth, or to a patient whose caloric demands are greater than his intake. Duodenal or jejunal feedings decrease the risk of aspiration because the formula bypasses the pylorus. Jejunal feedings reduce pancreatic stimulation; thus, may require an elemental diet. They're usually given on an intermittent schedule; patients getting duodenal or jejunal feedings typically better tolerate a continuous slow drip. Liquid nutrient solutions come in various formulas for administration through a nasogastric tube, small-bore feeding tube, gastrostomy or jejunostomy tube, percutaneous endoscopic gastrostomy or jejunostomy tube, or gastrostomy feeding button. A bulb syringe or large catheter-tip syringe may be substituted for a gavage bag if the patient tolerates a gravity drip infusion. The physician may order an infusion pump to ensure accurate delivery of the prescribed formula.

CONTRAINDICATIONS
▪ Absent bowel sounds
▪ Suspected intestinal obstruction

EQUIPMENT
For gastric feedings
Feeding formula ● graduated container ● 120 ml of water ● gavage bag with tubing and flow regulator clamp ● towel or linen-saver pad ● 60-ml syringe ● pH test strip ● adapter to connect gavage tubing to feeding tube ● infusion controller and tubing set (optional, for continuous administration)

For duodenal or jejunal feedings
Feeding formula ● enteral administration set containing a gavage container, drip chamber, roller clamp or flow regulator, and tube connector ● I.V. pole ● 60-ml syringe with adapter tip ● water ● Y connector ● pump administration set (optional, for an enteral infusion pump)

For nasal and oral care
Cotton-tipped applicators ● water-soluble lubricant ● sponge-tipped swabs ● petroleum jelly ● tape

PREPARATION OF EQUIPMENT
▪ Refrigerate any formulas prepared in the dietary department or pharmacy. Refrigerate commercial formulas only after opening them.

- Check the date on all formula containers. Discard expired formula.
- Use powdered formula within 24 hours of mixing.
- Shake the container well to mix thoroughly, and allow the formula to warm to room temperature before giving (never warm it over direct heat or in a microwave; heat may curdle the formula or change its chemical composition). Cold formula can increase the chance of diarrhea.
- Pour 60 ml of water into the graduated container.
- After closing the flow clamp on the administration set, pour the appropriate amount of formula into the gavage bag.
- To prevent bacterial growth, don't hang more than a 4- to 6-hour supply at one time.
- Open the flow clamp on the administration set to purge air from the tubing. This keeps air from entering the patient's stomach and causing distention.

ESSENTIAL STEPS

- Verify the patient's identity using two patient identifiers, such as the patient's name and identification number.
- Provide privacy and wash your hands.
- Inform the patient that he'll receive nourishment through the tube, and reinforce the explanation of the procedure. If possible, give him a schedule of subsequent feedings.
- If the patient has a nasal or oral tube, cover his chest with a towel or linen-saver pad to protect him and the bed linens from spills.
- Monitor for bowel sounds and abdominal distention.

Delivering a gastric feeding

- Elevate the bed to semi-Fowler's or high Fowler's position to prevent aspiration by gastroesophageal reflux, and to promote digestion.
- Confirm the placement of the feeding tube.

   RED FLAG Never give a tube feeding until you're sure the tube is properly positioned in his stomach; otherwise, it could cause formula to enter his lungs.
- To check tube patency and position, remove the cap or plug from the feeding tube and attach the syringe.
- Gently aspirate gastric secretions.
- Examine the aspirate and, if congruent with your facility's policy, place a small amount on the pH test strip. It's likely that the gastric tube is properly placed if the aspirate has a typical gastric fluid appearance (grassy-green, clear and colorless with mucus shreds, or brown) and the pH is 5.0 or less. For a truly accurate

pH reading, tube feedings should be held for 1 hour before the reading, if possible.

■ To monitor gastric emptying, aspirate and measure residual gastric contents. Withhold feedings if residual volume is greater than the predetermined amount specified in the physician's order (usually 50 to 100 ml). Reinstill aspirate obtained since it contains electrolytes.

■ Connect the gavage bag tubing to the feeding tube; you may need to use an adapter to connect the two.

■ If using a bulb or catheter-tip syringe, remove the bulb or plunger and attach the syringe to the pinched-off feeding tube to prevent excess air from entering the patient's stomach, causing distention.

■ Open the regulator clamp on the gavage bag tubing and adjust the infusion rate appropriately.

■ When using a bulb syringe, fill the syringe with formula and release the feeding tube to allow formula to flow through it. The height at which you hold the syringe will determine infusion rate. When the syringe is three-quarters empty, pour more formula into it.

■ To prevent air from entering the tube and the patient's stomach, never allow the syringe to empty completely.

■ If you're using an administration pump, set the infusion rate according to the physician's orders.

■ Always give a tube feeding slowly—typically 200 to 350 ml over 15 to 30 minutes, depending on the patient's tolerance and the physician's order—to prevent sudden stomach distention, which can cause nausea, vomiting, cramps, or diarrhea.

■ After giving the appropriate amount of formula, flush the tubing by adding about 60 ml of water to the gavage bag or bulb syringe, or manually flush it using a barrel syringe. This maintains the tube's patency by removing excess formula, which could occlude the tube.

■ If you're giving a continuous feeding, flush the feeding tube and monitor gastric emptying by measuring residual gastric contents before initiating the feedings and every 4 hours.

■ To discontinue gastric feeding (depending on the equipment), close the regulator clamp on the gavage bag tubing, disconnect the syringe from the feeding tube, or turn off the infusion controller.

■ Cover the end of the feeding tube with its plug or cap to prevent leakage and contamination.

■ Leave the patient in semi-Fowler's or high Fowler's position for at least 30 minutes.

■ Rinse reusable equipment with warm water; dry and store in a convenient place for the next feeding. Change equipment every 24 hours or according to facility policy.

Delivering a duodenal or jejunal feeding

■ Elevate the head of the bed and place the patient in low-Fowler's position.
■ Open the enteral administration set and hang the gavage container on the I.V. pole.
■ If using a nasoduodenal tube, measure its length to check tube placement. You may not get residual gastric contents when you aspirate the tube.
■ Open the flow clamp and regulate the flow to the desired rate.
■ To regulate the rate using a volumetric infusion pump, follow the manufacturer's directions and physician's orders for equipment setup. Most patients receive small amounts at first, with volumes increasing gradually when tolerance is established.
■ Flush the tube before feedings and every 4 hours with water to maintain patency and provide hydration. A needle catheter jejunostomy tube may require flushing every 2 hours to prevent formula buildup inside the tube.
■ A Y-connector may be useful for frequent flushing. Attach the continuous feeding to the main port and use the side port for flushes.
■ Change equipment every 24 hours or according to facility policy.

SPECIAL CONSIDERATIONS

■ If the feeding solution doesn't initially flow through a bulb syringe, attach the bulb and squeeze it gently to start the flow; then remove the bulb.
■ Never use the bulb to force formula through the tube.
■ If the patient becomes nauseated or vomits, stop feeding immediately. He may vomit if his stomach becomes distended from overfeeding or delayed gastric emptying.
■ To reduce oropharyngeal discomfort caused by the tube, allow him to brush his teeth or care for his dentures regularly and encourage frequent gargling.
■ If the patient is unconscious, give oral care with wet sponge-tipped swabs every 4 hours. Use petroleum jelly on dry, cracked lips.
■ Dry mucous membranes may indicate dehydration, which requires increased fluid intake.

- Clean the patient's nostrils with cotton-tipped applicators, apply water-soluble lubricant along the mucosa, and monitor the skin for signs of breakdown.
- During continuous feedings, monitor the patient frequently for abdominal distention. Flush the tubing by adding about 50 ml of water to the gavage bag or bulb syringe. This maintains the tube's patency by removing excess formula, which can occlude the tube.
- If the patient develops diarrhea, give small, frequent, less concentrated feedings, or give bolus feedings over a longer time.
- Make sure the formula isn't cold and proper storage and sanitation practices have been followed.
- Loose stools associated with tube feedings make extra perineal and skin care necessary. Giving paregoric, tincture of opium, or diphenoxylate hydrochloride as prescribed, may improve the condition; changing to a formula with more fiber may eliminate liquid stools.

RED FLAG *Send a stool specimen for culture before starting antidiarrheal drugs.*

- If the patient is constipated, the physician may change the formula.
- Monitor the patient's hydration status; increase fluid intake as ordered. If the condition persists, give an appropriate drug or enema, as ordered.
- Drugs can be given through the feeding tube; however, some drugs may change the osmolarity of the feeding formula and cause diarrhea.
- Except for enteric-coated drugs or time-released drugs, crush tablets or open and dilute capsules in water before giving them. Be sure to flush the tubing afterward to ensure full instillation of the drug.
- Small-bore feeding tubes may kink, making instillation impossible. Change the patient's position or notify the physician to withdraw the tube a few inches and restart.

RED FLAG *Never use a guide wire to reposition the tube; it may puncture the tube and perforate the stomach or intestine.*

- Constantly monitor the infusion rate of a blended or high-residue formula to determine if the formula is clogging the tubing as it settles. To prevent such clogging, squeeze the bag frequently throughout the feeding to agitate the solution.
- Collect blood samples as ordered.
- Glycosuria, hyperglycemia, and diuresis can indicate an excessive carbohydrate level, leading to hyperosmotic dehydration, which may be fatal.

■ Check blood glucose levels to monitor glucose tolerance.
■ Monitor electrolytes, blood urea nitrogen, glucose, and osmolality to determine response to therapy and monitor hydration status.
■ Check the infusion rate hourly to ensure correct infusion. (With an improvised administration set, use a time tape to record the rate because it's difficult to get precise readings from an irrigation container or enema bag.)
■ For duodenal or jejunal feeding, most patients tolerate a continuous drip better than bolus feedings, which can cause hyperglycemia and diarrhea.
■ Until the patient tolerates the formula, you may need to dilute it to one-half or three-quarters strength to start and increase it gradually, as ordered.

RED FLAG *Patients under stress or receiving steroids may experience a pseudodiabetic state. Monitor bedside blood glucose levels and report high levels; the physician may order insulin.*

■ Reinforce teaching about how to program and use the infusion control device, the use of the syringe or bag and tubing, the care of the tube and insertion site, and formula-mixing.
■ Remind the patient that the formula may be mixed in an electric blender according to package directions.
■ Reinforce that formula not used within 24 hours must be discarded. If the formula must hang for more than 8 hours, tell him to use a gavage or pump administration set with an ice pouch to decrease the incidence of bacterial growth.
■ Remind the patient to use a new bag daily.
■ Reinforce with family members the signs and symptoms to report to the physician or home care nurse, as well as measures to take in an emergency.

COMPLICATIONS

■ Complications include erosion of esophageal, tracheal, nasal, and oropharyngeal mucosa; bloating and retention when using the gastric route for frequent or large-volume feedings; dehydration, diarrhea, and vomiting, causing metabolic disturbances; a clogged feeding tube when using duodenal or jejunal route; metabolic, fluid, and electrolyte abnormalities including hyperglycemia, hyperosmolar dehydration, coma, edema, hypernatremia, and essential fatty acid deficiency; and dumping syndrome. (See *Managing tube feeding problems*.)
■ Cramping and abdominal distention usually indicate intolerance.

Managing tube feeding problems

COMPLICATIONS	NURSING INTERVENTIONS
Suspected aspiration of gastric secretions	• Discontinue feeding immediately. • Perform tracheal suction of aspirated contents if possible. • Notify the physician. Prophylactic antibiotics and chest physiotherapy may be ordered. • Check tube placement before feeding to prevent complication. • Keep the head of the bed elevated to at least 30 degrees during feedings.
Tube obstruction	• Flush the tube with warm water. If necessary, assist the physician to replace the tube. • Flush the tube with 50 ml of water after each feeding to remove excess formula, which could occlude the tube.
Oral, nasal, or pharyngeal irritation or necrosis	• Provide frequent oral hygiene using mouthwash or sponge-tipped swabs. Use petroleum jelly on cracked lips. • Change the tube's position. If necessary, assist the physician to replace the tube.
Vomiting, bloating, diarrhea, or cramps	• Reduce the flow rate or temporarily discontinue the feedings. • Administer metoclopramide as ordered to increase GI motility. • Warm the formula to prevent GI distress. • For 30 minutes after feeding, position the patient on his right side with his head elevated to facilitate gastric emptying. • Notify the physician. He may want to reduce the amount of formula being given during each feeding.
Constipation	• Provide additional fluids if the patient can tolerate them. • Administer a bulk-forming laxative. • Notify the physician. He may change the formula.
Electrolyte imbalance	• Monitor serum electrolyte levels. • Notify the physician. He may want to adjust the formula content to correct the deficiency.
Hyperglycemia	• Monitor blood glucose levels. • Notify the physician of elevated levels. • Administer insulin if ordered. • The physician may adjust the formula content.

DOCUMENTATION

- On the intake and output sheet, record the date and time and the volumes and types of formula and volume of water administered.
- In your notes, record a description of the patient's GI status (including tube exit site, if appropriate); amount of residual gastric contents; verification of tube placement; and tube patency.
- Note the patient's tolerance as well as any nausea, vomiting, cramping, diarrhea, and distention.
- Document drugs given through the tube.
- Record the date and time of administration set changes, oral and nasal hygiene, and results of blood and urine specimen collections.
- Note a description of the patient's hydration status.
- Document reinforced patient teaching and the patient's response.

8

GENITOURINARY CARE

The renal and urologic systems produce, transport, collect, and excrete urine. Dysfunctions in these systems impair fluid, electrolyte, and acid-base balance, as well as the elimination of waste. To restore or facilitate effective function of these systems, treatment of renal and urologic disorders usually involves temporary or permanent insertion of a urinary, peritoneal, or vascular catheter or tube. Catheterization also allows for monitoring of renal and urologic systems and aids in diagnosing the dysfunction. Nursing care focuses on providing catheter or tube care, monitoring output, and monitoring the patency of the catheter or tube. It also focuses on helping the patient to perform self-care when he will have the catheter in place long-term.

Arteriovenous shunt care

An arteriovenous (AV) shunt consists of two segments of tubing, joined in a U shape, that divert blood from an artery to a vein. A shunt is one way to provide access to the circulatory system for hemodialysis. (See *Hemodialysis access sites,* page 218.)

The device is usually inserted surgically in the forearm or (rarely) the ankle. After insertion, a shunt requires regular monitoring to ensure patency and monitoring of the surrounding skin for infection. Nursing care also includes aseptically cleaning arterial and venous exit sites, applying antiseptic ointment, and dressing sites with sterile bandages. When done just before hemodialysis, care prolongs the life of a shunt, helps prevent infection, and allows early detection of clotting. Shunt site care is done more often if the dressing becomes wet or nonocclusive.

CONTRAINDICATIONS
- Absence of radial artery pulsation
- Signs of infection

Hemodialysis access sites

Hemodialysis requires vascular access. The site and type of access may vary, depending on the expected duration of dialysis, the surgeon's preference, and the patient's condition.

SUBCLAVIAN VEIN CATHETERIZATION

Using the Seldinger technique, the physician or surgeon inserts an introducer needle into the subclavian vein. He then inserts a guide wire through the introducer needle and removes the needle. Using the guide wire, he then threads a 5″ to 12″ (12- to 30-cm) plastic or Teflon catheter (with a Y hub) into the patient's vein.

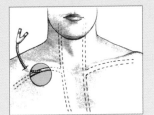

FEMORAL VEIN CATHETERIZATION

Using the Seldinger technique, the physician or surgeon inserts an introducer needle into the left or right femoral vein. He then inserts a guide wire through the introducer needle and removes the needle.

   Using the guide wire, he then threads a 5″ to 12″ plastic or Teflon catheter with a Y hub or two catheters, one for inflow and another placed about ½″ (1.3 cm) distal to the first for outflow.

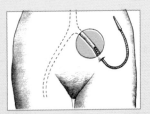

ARTERIOVENOUS FISTULA

To create a fistula, the surgeon makes an incision into the patient's wrist or lower forearm, then a small incision in the side of an artery and another in the side of a vein. He sutures the edges of the incisions together to make a common opening 3 to 7 mm long.

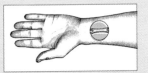

Hemodialysis access sites *(continued)*

ARTERIOVENOUS SHUNT
To create a shunt, the surgeon makes an incision in the patient's wrist, lower forearm, or (rarely) ankle. He then inserts a 6" to 10" (15- to 25-cm) transparent Silastic cannula into an artery and another into a vein. Finally, he tunnels the cannulas out through stab wounds and joins them with a piece of Teflon tubing.

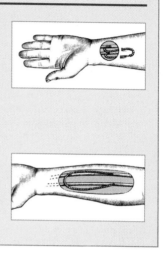

ARTERIOVENOUS GRAFT
To create a graft, the surgeon makes an incision in the patient's forearm, upper arm, or thigh. He then tunnels a natural or synthetic graft under the skin and sutures the distal end to an artery and the proximal end to a vein.

EQUIPMENT

Drape ● stethoscope ● sterile gloves ● sterile 4" × 4" gauze pads ● sterile cotton-tipped applicators ● antiseptic (usually povidone-iodine solution) ● bulldog clamps ● plasticized or hypoallergenic tape ● swab specimen kit (optional) ● prescribed antimicrobial ointment (usually povidone-iodine) ● sterile elastic gauze bandage ● 2" × 2" gauze pads ● hydrogen peroxide ● prepackaged kits are available

ESSENTIAL STEPS

- Verify the patient's identity using two patient identifiers, such as the patient's name and identification number.
- Reinforce the explanation of the procedure to the patient.
- Provide privacy and wash your hands.
- Place a drape on a stable surface, such as a bedside table, to reduce risk of traumatic injury to the shunt site.
- Place the shunted extremity on a draped surface.
- Remove the two bulldog clamps from the elastic gauze bandage and unwrap the bandage from the shunt area.
- Carefully remove gauze dressing covering the shunt and the 4" × 4" gauze pad under the shunt.

■ Monitor arterial and venous exit sites for signs and symptoms of infection, such as erythema, swelling, excessive tenderness, or drainage.

■ Obtain a swab specimen of purulent drainage and tell the physician immediately about signs of infection.

■ Check blood flow through the shunt by inspecting the color of the blood (it should be bright red) and comparing the warmth of the shunt with that of surrounding skin (it should feel as warm as the skin).

RED FLAG If blood is dark purple or black and the temperature of the shunt is lower than the surrounding skin, the shunt has clotted. Notify the physician immediately.

RED FLAG To prevent shunt occlusion, avoid blood pressure measurement and venipuncture in the affected arm.

■ Clean a stethoscope and use it to auscultate the shunt between the arterial and venous exit sites. A bruit confirms normal blood flow.

■ Don't use a Doppler device to auscultate because it will detect peripheral blood flow as well as shunt-related sounds.

■ Palpate the shunt for a thrill (by lightly placing fingertips over access site and feeling for vibration), which also shows normal blood flow.

■ Open a few 4″ × 4″ gauze pads and cotton-tipped applicators, and soak them with antiseptic.

■ Put on sterile gloves.

■ Clean skin at one of the exit sites using a 4″ × 4″ gauze pad.

■ Wipe away from the site to remove bacteria and prevent contamination of the shunt.

■ Use the soaked cotton-tipped applicators to remove crusted material from the exit site; encrustations enable bacterial growth.

■ Clean the other exit site using fresh, soaked 4″ × 4″ gauze pads and cotton-tipped applicators.

■ Clean the rest of the skin that was covered by gauze dressing with fresh, soaked 4″ × 4″ gauze pads.

■ Apply antimicrobial ointment to the exit sites to prevent infection, if ordered.

■ Place a dry, sterile 4″ × 4″ gauze pad under the shunt to prevent it from contacting skin, which could cause irritation and breakdown.

■ Cover exit sites with dry, sterile 4″ × 4″ gauze pads; to keep exit sites clean and protected, tape gauze pads securely.

■ For daily care, wrap shunt with an elastic gauze bandage.

■ Leave a small part of the shunt cannula exposed so the patient can check for patency without removing the dressing.

- Place bulldog clamps on the edge of the elastic gauze bandage so the patient can use them to stop hemorrhage in case the shunt separates.
- Follow facility procedure for shunt separation.
- For care before hemodialysis, don't redress the shunt, but keep bulldog clamps accessible.

SPECIAL CONSIDERATIONS

- Make sure the AV junction of the shunt is secured with plasticized or hypoallergenic tape to prevent separation of the two halves of the shunt and minimize risk of hemorrhage.
- Handle the shunt and dressings carefully.

   RED FLAG Don't use sharp instruments or scissors to remove the dressing because you may cut the shunt, and never remove the tape securing the AV junction during dressing changes.
- Use each 4″ × 4″ gauze pad only once when cleaning shunt exit sites.
- Make sure the tape doesn't kink or occlude the shunt when redressing the site.
- If the exit sites are heavily encrusted, place a 2″ × 2″ hydrogen peroxide–soaked gauze pad on the area for about 1 hour to loosen crust.
- Make sure the patient isn't allergic to iodine before using povidone-iodine solution or ointment.
- Make sure the patient knows how to care for the shunt; reinforce proper home care, if necessary.

COMPLICATIONS

None known.

DOCUMENTATION

- Note that shunt care was given.
- Describe the condition of the shunt and surrounding skin.
- Note the ointment used.
- Document reinforced patient teaching.
- Record the presence of a bruit and thrill, the color of the blood in the shunt, and the temperature of the site.

Bladder ultrasonography

Urine retention, a potentially life-threatening condition, may result from neurologic or psychological disorders or obstruction of urine flow. Medications such as anticholinergics, antihistamines, and antidepressants may also cause urine retention. Urinary catheterization, the traditional method for measuring urine volume in the bladder, places the patient at risk for infection. Noninvasive bladder ultrasonography, however, provides an accurate measurement of urine volume with reduced risk of urinary tract infection.

CONTRAINDICATIONS

None known.

EQUIPMENT

BladderScan (ultrasound) unit with scanhead ● ultrasonic transmission gel ● alcohol pad washcloth ● gloves

ESSENTIAL STEPS

■ Bring the ultrasound unit to the bedside. Verify the patient's identity using two patient identifiers, such as the patient's name and identification number. Reinforce the explanation of the procedure to the patient to help reduce his anxiety.

■ Choose the appropriate gender setting (male or female), since the uterus resembles the bladder. For a female patient who has had a hysterectomy in the past, choose the male gender setting.

■ Wash your hands and provide privacy.

■ If this is a postvoiding scan, ask the patient to void. Position the patient in a supine position.

■ Put on gloves and clean the rounded end of the scanhead with an alcohol pad.

■ Expose the patient's suprapubic area.

■ Turn on the ultrasound by pressing the button (designated by a dot within a circle) on the far left and press scan.

■ Place ultrasonic gel on the scanhead to promote an airtight seal for optimal sound-wave transmission.

■ Tell the patient that the gel will feel cold when placed on the abdomen. Locate the symphysis pubis, and place the scanhead about 1″ (2.5 cm) superior to the symphysis pubis.

■ Locate the icon (a rough figure of a person) on the probe and make sure the head of the icon points toward the head of the patient.

■ Press the scanhead button marked with a sound wave pattern to activate the scan. Hold the scanhead steady until a beep sounds.

■ Look at the aiming icon and screen, which displays the bladder position and volume. Reposition the probe, and scan until the bladder is centered in the aiming screen. The largest measurement will be saved.

■ Press "Done" when finished.

- The ultrasound will display the measured urine volume and the longitudinal and horizontal axis scans.
- Press "Print" to obtain a hard copy of your results.
- Turn off the ultrasound. Use a disinfecting solution to clean the gel off the scanhead.
- Use a washcloth to remove the gel from the patient's skin.
- Remove your gloves and wash your hands.

SPECIAL CONSIDERATIONS

- Report the results to the physician. Depending on the volume of urine in the bladder, he may order the patient to be catheterized.
- Reinforce that the patient needs to remain supine and as still as possible to obtain an accurate reading.

COMPLICATIONS

None known.

DOCUMENTATION

- Document whether the patient voided before the scan was performed.
- Record the patient's name, the date, and the time of the scan on the printout and attach it to the patient's medical record.
- Document the urine volume, as well as any treatment, in the patient's medical record.

Catheter irrigation

To avoid introducing microorganisms into the bladder, urinary catheter irrigation is only done to remove an obstruction such as a blood clot that develops after bladder, kidney, or prostate surgery.

CONTRAINDICATIONS

Use caution if the patient has recently had prostate, bladder, ureteral, or kidney surgery. Contact the physician; he may want to perform the irrigation himself.

EQUIPMENT

Ordered irrigating solution (such as normal saline solution) ● sterile graduated receptacle or emesis basin ● sterile bulb syringe or 60-ml catheter tip syringe ● two alcohol pads ● sterile gloves ● linen-saver pad ● intake-output sheet ● basin of warm water (optional)

PREPARATION OF EQUIPMENT

■ Check the expiration date on the irrigating solution and warm the solution to room temperature to prevent vesical spasms during instillation.

■ If necessary, place the container in a basin of warm water.

■ Wash your hands and assemble the equipment at the bedside.

RED FLAG *Never heat the solution on a burner or in a microwave. Hot irrigating solution can injure the patient's bladder.*

ESSENTIAL STEPS

■ Verify the patient's identity using two patient identifiers, such as the patient's name and identification number.

■ Reinforce the explanation of the procedure to the patient and provide privacy.

■ Place the patient in dorsal recumbent position.

■ Place a linen-saver pad under the patient's buttocks to protect bed linens.

■ Create a sterile field at the patient's bedside by opening the sterile equipment tray or commercial kit.

■ Clean the lip of the solution bottle by pouring a small amount into a sink or waste receptacle, using sterile technique.

■ Pour the prescribed amount of solution into the graduated receptacle or emesis basin.

■ Place the tip of the syringe into the solution.

■ Squeeze the bulb or pull back the plunger (depending on type of syringe) and fill the syringe with appropriate amount of solution (usually 30 ml).

■ Open the package of alcohol pads and put on sterile gloves.

■ Clean the juncture of the catheter and drainage tube with an alcohol pad to remove as many bacterial contaminants as possible.

■ Disconnect the catheter and drainage tube by twisting them in opposite directions and carefully pulling them apart without creating tension on the catheter.

■ Don't let go of the catheter—hold it in your nondominant hand.

■ Place the end of the drainage tube on the sterile field, making sure not to contaminate it.

■ Keep the end of the drainage tube sterile by placing sterile gauze over it and securing the gauze with a piece of tape.

■ Twist the bulb syringe or catheter-tip syringe onto the catheter's distal end.

■ Squeeze the bulb or slowly push the plunger of the syringe to instill the irrigating solution through the catheter.

- Refill the syringe and repeat this step until you've instilled the prescribed amount of irrigating solution, if necessary.
- Remove the syringe and direct the return flow from the catheter into a graduated receptacle or emesis basin.
- Don't let the catheter end touch the drainage in the receptacle or become contaminated in any way.
- Wipe the end of the drainage tube and catheter with the remaining alcohol pad.
- Wait a few seconds until the alcohol evaporates; then reattach the drainage tubing to the catheter.
- Dispose of all used supplies properly.

SPECIAL CONSIDERATIONS
- Catheter irrigation requires strict sterile technique to prevent bacteria from entering the bladder.
- The ends of the catheter and drainage tube and tip of the syringe must be kept sterile throughout procedure.

RED FLAG If you encounter resistance during instillation of irrigating solution, don't try to force the solution into the bladder. Instead, stop the procedure and notify the physician.

RED FLAG If an indwelling catheter becomes totally obstructed, obtain an order to remove it and replace it with a new one to prevent bladder distention, acute renal failure, urinary stasis, and subsequent infection.

- The physician may order a continuous irrigation system, which decreases risk of infection by eliminating the need to disconnect the catheter and drainage tube repeatedly.
- Encourage patients not on restricted fluid intake to increase intake to 3,000 ml per day to help flush the urinary system and reduce sediment formation.
- To keep the patient's urine acidic and help prevent calculus formation, tell him to eat foods containing ascorbic acid, including citrus fruits and juices, cranberry juice, and dark green and deep yellow vegetables.
- Reinforce that the patient remain as still as possible and should report any discomfort during the procedure.

COMPLICATIONS
Introduction of bacteria into the urinary tract can produce a urinary tract infection.

DOCUMENTATION

- Note the amount, color, and consistency of return urine flow, and document the patient's tolerance of the procedure.
- Note resistance during instillation of the solution.
- If the return flow volume is less than the amount of solution instilled, note this on the intake and output balance sheets and in your notes.

Continuous bladder irrigation

Continuous bladder irrigation helps prevent urinary tract obstruction by flushing out small blood clots that form after prostate or bladder surgery. It can be used to prevent and treat an irritated, inflamed, or infected bladder lining. Continuous flow of irrigating solution through the bladder creates a mild tamponade that may help prevent venous hemorrhage. (See *Setup for continuous bladder irrigation.*)

The catheter is usually inserted during prostate or bladder surgery but may be inserted at the bedside for a nonsurgical patient.

CONTRAINDICATIONS

None known.

EQUIPMENT

One 4,000-ml container or two 2,000-ml containers of irrigating solution (usually normal saline solution) or prescribed amount of medicated solution ● Y-type tubing made specifically for bladder irrigation ● alcohol or povidone-iodine pad

PREPARATION OF EQUIPMENT

- Assemble all equipment at the patient's bedside.
- Use Y-type tubing to allow immediate irrigation with reserve solution.
- Large volumes of irrigating solution are usually required during the first 24 to 48 hours after surgery.
- Before starting, double-check the irrigating solution against the physician's order.
- If the solution contains an antibiotic, check the patient's chart to make sure he isn't allergic to the drug.

ESSENTIAL STEPS

- Verify the patient's identity using two patient identifiers, such as the patient's name and identification number.

Setup for continuous bladder irrigation

In continuous bladder irrigation, a triple-lumen catheter allows irrigating solution to flow into the bladder through one lumen and flow out through another. The third lumen is used to inflate the balloon that holds the catheter in place.

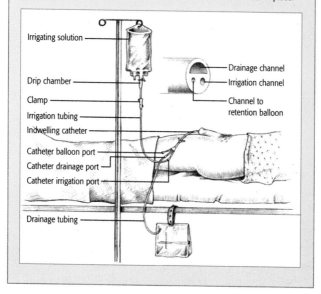

- The patient should remain on bed rest throughout continuous bladder irrigation, unless specified otherwise.
- Wash your hands.
- Reinforce the explanation of the procedure and provide privacy.
- Insert the spike of the Y-type tubing into the container of irrigating solution.
- With a two-container system, insert one spike into each container.
- Squeeze the drip chamber on the spike of the tubing.
- Open the flow clamp and purge the tubing to remove air which could cause bladder distention.
- Close the clamp.
- Hang the bag, or bags, of irrigating solution on the I.V. pole.

■ Clean the opening to the inflow lumen of the catheter with the alcohol or povidone-iodine pad.
■ Insert the distal end of the Y-type tubing securely into the inflow lumen (third port) of the catheter.
■ Make sure the catheter's outflow lumen is securely attached to the drainage bag tubing.
■ Open the flow clamp under the container of irrigating solution and set the drip rate as ordered.
■ Secure the catheter to the patient's leg with tape or a leg band.
■ To prevent air from entering the system, don't allow the primary container to empty completely before replacing it.
■ If you have a two-container system, simultaneously close the flow clamp under the nearly empty container and open the flow clamp under the reserve container. This prevents reflux of irrigating solution from the reserve container into the nearly empty one.
■ Hang a new reserve container on the I.V. pole and insert the tubing, maintaining asepsis.
■ Empty the drainage bag about every 4 hours or as often as needed.
■ Use sterile technique to avoid risk of contamination.
■ Monitor vital signs at least every 4 hours during irrigation, increasing the frequency if the patient becomes unstable.
■ Monitor for bladder distention, catheter leaking, and bladder spasms.

SPECIAL CONSIDERATIONS
■ Check inflow and outflow lines periodically for kinks to make sure the solution is running freely.
■ If the physician has ordered that the solution flow rapidly, check the lines frequently.
■ Measure outflow volume accurately (every 10 to 15 minutes for the first 1 to 2 hours and then as needed or as ordered, usually hourly).
■ Outflow should be the same or slightly more than inflow volume, allowing for urine production.

RED FLAG Postoperative inflow volume exceeding outflow volume may indicate bladder rupture at the suture lines or renal damage; notify the physician immediately.

■ Monitor the outflow for changes in appearance (color and clarity) and for blood clots, especially if irrigation is being done postoperatively to control bleeding.

⚑ **RED FLAG** *If the drainage is bright red, irrigating solution should be infused rapidly with the clamp wide open until drainage clears. Notify the physician immediately if you suspect hemorrhage.*

■ If the drainage is clear, the solution is usually given at a rate of 40 to 60 drops/minute.
■ The physician usually specifies the rate for antibiotic solutions.
■ Encourage oral fluid intake of 2 to 3 qt (2 to 3 L)/day unless contraindicated.
■ Reinforce that the patient must remain on bed rest during the treatment, unless otherwise ordered.
■ Reinforce the explanation of the procedure. Remind the patient to report symptoms such as pain or bladder distention.

COMPLICATIONS
Complications include infection caused by interruptions in a continuous irrigation system and bladder distention and spasms caused by obstruction in the catheter's outflow lumen.

DOCUMENTATION
■ Each time a container of solution is finished, record the date, time, and amount of fluid administered and drained on the intake and output record.
■ Record the time and amount of fluid each time you empty the drainage bag.
■ Note the appearance of the drainage and patient complaints.

Indwelling catheter care and removal

Urinary catheter care is intended to prevent infection and other complications by keeping the catheter and insertion sites clean. Care is performed daily after the patient's morning bath and right after perineal care. Bedtime care may be performed before perineal care. The equipment and the patient's genitalia require inspection at least twice daily.

The catheter is removed when bladder decompression is no longer needed, when the patient can resume voiding, or when the catheter is obstructed. The physician may order bladder retraining before catheter removal, depending on the length of time of catheterization. Some facilities don't recommend daily care because of the increased risk of infection and other complications. Become familiar with facility policy.

CONTRAINDICATIONS
None known.

EQUIPMENT
For urinary catheter care
Soap and water ● sterile gloves ● eight sterile 4″ × 4″ gauze pads ● basin or basins ● washcloth ● leg bag ● collection bag ● adhesive tape or leg band ● waste receptacle ● optional: safety pin, rubber band, gooseneck lamp or flashlight, adhesive remover, and specimen container

For perineal cleaning
Washcloth ● additional basin ● soap and water

For urinary catheter removal
Gloves ● alcohol pad ● 10-ml syringe with a Luer-Lok ● bedpan ● linen-saver pad ● clamp for bladder retraining (optional)

PREPARATION OF EQUIPMENT
■ Wash your hands and bring the equipment to the bedside.
■ Open the gauze pads, place several in the first basin, and pour povidone-iodine or other cleaning agent over them.

>   *RED FLAG Some facilities specify that after wiping the urinary meatus with cleaning solution, you should wipe it off with wet, sterile gauze pads to prevent irritation from the cleaning solution. If this is a requirement at your facility, pour water into second basin and moisten three more gauze pads.*

ESSENTIAL STEPS
■ Verify the patient's identity using two patient identifiers, such as the patient's name and identification number.
■ Reinforce the explanation of the procedure and its purpose to the patient.
■ Provide privacy.

Urinary catheter care
■ Make sure lighting is adequate so you can see the perineum and catheter tubing clearly. Place a lamp or flashlight at the bedside if needed.
■ Inspect the catheter for problems and monitor urine drainage for mucus, blood clots, sediment, and turbidity.

>   *RED FLAG If you notice mucus, blood clots, sediment, or turbidity in the urine drainage or lumen (or if your facility's policy*

requires it), obtain a sterile urine specimen (collect at least 3 ml of urine, but don't fill the specimen cup more than halfway) and notify the physician.

■ Pinch the catheter between two fingers to determine if the lumen contains any material.

■ Monitor the outside of the catheter where it enters the urinary meatus for encrusted material and suppurative drainage.

■ Monitor the tissue around the meatus for irritation or swelling.

■ Remove the leg band or adhesive tape used to secure the catheter.

■ Inspect the area for signs and symptoms of adhesive burns—redness, tenderness, or blisters.

■ Put on gloves.

■ Clean the outside of the catheter and tissue around the meatus, using soap and water.

🚩 **RED FLAG** *To avoid contaminating the urinary tract, always clean by wiping away from—never toward—the urinary meatus, in a downward motion toward the rectal area.*

■ Use a dry gauze pad to remove encrusted material.

🚩 **RED FLAG** *Don't pull on the catheter while cleaning it. This can injure the urethra and bladder wall. It can also expose a section of the catheter that was inside the urethra; when you release the catheter the newly contaminated section will reenter the urethra, introducing potentially infectious organisms.*

■ Remove your gloves, reapply the leg band, and reattach the catheter to the leg band.

■ If a leg band isn't available, use adhesive tape.

■ To prevent skin hypersensitivity or irritation, retape the catheter on the opposite side.

🚩 **RED FLAG** *Provide enough slack before securing the catheter to prevent tension on the tubing, which could injure the urethral lumen or bladder wall.*

■ Most drainage bags have a plastic clamp on the tubing to attach them to the sheet. If a plastic clamp isn't provided, wrap a rubber band around the drainage tubing, insert the safety pin through a loop of the rubber band and pin the tubing to the sheet below bladder level.

■ Attach the collection bag, below bladder level, to the bed frame.

■ Clean residue from the previous tape site with adhesive remover, if necessary.

■ Dispose of all used supplies in a waste receptacle.

Urinary catheter removal

■ Confirm the physician's order to remove the catheter.

- Wash your hands.
- Assemble equipment at the patient's bedside.
- Reinforce the explanation of the procedure and tell the patient he may feel slight discomfort or a burning sensation.
- Remind the patient that voiding usually resumes within 8 hours after catheter removal and that you'll check periodically during the first 6 to 24 hours to make sure he resumes voiding.
- Put on gloves.
- Place a linen-saver pad under the patient's buttocks.
- Attach the syringe to the Luer-Lock mechanism on the catheter.
- Pull back on the plunger of the syringe to deflate the balloon by aspirating the injected fluid.
- The amount of fluid injected is usually indicated on the tip of the catheter's balloon lumen and recorded on the care plan or Kardex and the patient's chart.
- Offer the patient a bedpan because urine may leak as the catheter is removed.
- Grasp the catheter and pinch it firmly with your thumb and index finger to prevent urine from flowing back into the urethra.
- Gently pull the catheter from the urethra.
- If there's resistance, don't apply force. Make sure that the balloon is completely deflated by attaching a new syringe to the balloon lumen of the catheter and pulling back. If it's deflated, notify the physician.
- Remove the bedpan, keeping it in easy reach and clear the path to the bathroom. Provide a urinal to a male patient.
- Measure and record the amount of urine in the collection bag before discarding.
- Remove and discard gloves, and wash your hands.
- After catheter removal, note the time and amount of each voiding.

SPECIAL CONSIDERATIONS
- Your facility may require the use of specific cleaning agents for urinary catheter care; check policy before beginning procedure.
- A physician's order will be needed to apply antibiotic ointments to the urinary meatus after cleaning.
- Avoid raising the drainage bag above bladder level to prevent reflux of urine, which may contain bacteria.
- To avoid damaging the urethral lumen or bladder wall, disconnect the drainage bag and tubing from the bed linen and bed frame before helping the patient out of bed.
- When possible, attach a leg bag to allow him greater mobility.

- If the patient will be discharged with an indwelling urinary catheter, reinforce teaching about how to use a leg bag.
- Encourage patients with unrestricted fluid intake to increase intake to at least 3 qt (3 L)/day to help flush the urinary system and reduce sediment formation.
- To prevent urinary sediment and calculi from obstructing the drainage tube, some patients are placed on an acid-ash diet to acidify the urine.
- After catheter removal, report incidents of incontinence (or dribbling), urgency, persistent dysuria or bladder spasms, fever, chills, or palpable bladder distention.
- When changing a catheter after long-term use (usually 30 days), you may need a larger catheter because the meatus enlarges, causing urine to leak around the catheter.
- Remind the patient discharged with an indwelling urinary catheter to wash the urinary meatus and perineal area with soap and water twice daily and the anal area after each bowel movement.

COMPLICATIONS

Complications may develop if the patient isn't kept well hydrated. Monitor for bladder discomfort or distention. Urinary tract infection may occur. Signs and symptoms include cloudy or foul smelling urine, hematuria, fever, malaise, tenderness over bladder, and flank pain. Failure of the balloon to deflate and rupture of the balloon may occur during removal.

RED FLAG Be alert for sharply reduced urine flow from the catheter. Acute renal failure may result from a catheter obstructed by sediment.

DOCUMENTATION

- Record care performed, modifications, patient complaints, and the condition of the perineum and urinary meatus.
- Note the character of the urine in the drainage bag.
- Report sediment buildup.
- Note whether a specimen was sent for laboratory analysis and the results.
- Record fluid intake and output.
- Provide an hourly record (usually necessary) for critically ill patients and those with renal insufficiency who are hemodynamically unstable.

- For bladder retraining, record the date and time the catheter was clamped, the time it was released, and the volume and appearance of urine.
- For urinary catheter removal, record the date and time and the patient's tolerance of the procedure.
- Report when and how much the patient voided after the catheter was removed and associated problems.

Indwelling catheter insertion

An indwelling catheter, also known as a *Foley or retention catheter,* remains in the bladder to provide continuous urine drainage. A balloon inflated at the catheter's distal end prevents it from slipping out of the bladder after insertion. Urinary catheters are most commonly used to relieve bladder distention caused by urine retention; to allow continuous urine drainage when the urinary meatus is swollen from childbirth, surgery, or local trauma: and after surgery to ensure adequate hourly urine production. They're also used to treat urinary tract obstruction (by a tumor or enlarged prostate), urine retention or infection from a neurogenic bladder caused by spinal cord injury or disease, and illness in which the patient's urine output must be monitored closely. They're used during bladder retraining for patients with neurologic disorders, such as stroke or spinal cord injury, to determine post-void residual urine volume and the need for intermittent catheterization. An indwelling urinary catheter is inserted only when absolutely necessary. Insertion should be performed with extreme care and sterile technique to prevent injury and infection.

CONTRAINDICATIONS

If the patient has a history of benign prosthetic hyperplasia or has had a recent prostate or urethral surgery or kidney transplant, contact the physician before inserting a catheter. The physician may want to perform it himself or may want the catheter inserted under cystoscopy.

EQUIPMENT

Sterile indwelling urinary catheter (preferably silicone #10 to #22 French [average adult sizes #16 to #18 French] or latex) ● syringe filled with 5 to 8 ml of sterile water ● washcloth ● towel ● soap and water ● two linen-saver pads ● sterile gloves ● sterile drape ● sterile fenestrated drape ● sterile cotton-tipped applicators (or cotton balls and plastic forceps) ● povidone-iodine or other antiseptic cleaning agent ● urine receptacle ● sterile water-soluble lubricant ● sterile

drainage collection bag ● intake and output sheet ● adhesive tape ●
urine-specimen container and laboratory request form, leg band
with Velcro closure, gooseneck lamp or flashlight, pillows or rolled
blankets or towels (optional)

PREPARATION OF EQUIPMENT

■ Confirm the order on the patient's chart and determine if the
catheter size or type has been specified.
■ Wash your hands.
■ Select appropriate equipment and assemble it at the patient's bedside.

ESSENTIAL STEPS

■ Verify the patient's identity using two patient identifiers, such as
the patient's name and identification number.
■ Reinforce the explanation of the procedure to the patient and
provide privacy.
■ Check the patient's chart and ask when he voided last.
■ Monitor the patient's genitourinary status.
■ Ask the patient whether he feels the urge to void.
■ In poor lighting, have a coworker hold a flashlight, use the overhead examination light, or place a lamp next to the patient's bed
so you can see the urinary meatus clearly.
■ Place the female patient in a supine position, with her knees
flexed and separated and her feet flat on the bed, about 2′ (61
cm) apart.
■ If she finds this position uncomfortable, have her flex one knee
and keep the other leg flat on the bed, ask her to lie on her side
with her knees drawn up to her chest, or place the soles of her
feet together and flex her knees during the catheterization procedure. These positions may be especially helpful for elderly, dis-
abled, or orthopedic patients or for patients with severe contractures.

RED FLAG Elderly patients may need pillows, rolled towels, or
blankets to provide positioning support.

■ Get assistance as needed to help the patient stay in position or to
direct light.
■ Place the male patient in a supine position with legs extended
and flat on the bed.
■ Ask the patient to hold the position to give a clear view of the
urinary meatus and prevent contamination of the sterile field.
■ Use the washcloth to clean the patient's genital area and perineum thoroughly with soap and water.

- Dry the area with the towel.
- Wash your hands.
- Place the linen-saver pads on the bed between the patient's legs and under the hips.
- To create a sterile field, open the prepackaged kit or equipment tray and place it between the female patient's legs or next to the male patient's hip.
- If sterile gloves are the first item on the tray, put them on.
- Place the sterile drape under the patient's hips.
- Drape the patient's lower abdomen with the sterile fenestrated drape so only the genital area remains exposed.
- Take care not to contaminate your gloves.
- Open the rest of the kit or tray and put on sterile gloves if you haven't already.
- Tear open the packet of povidone-iodine or antiseptic cleaning agent and saturate sterile cotton balls or applicators, being careful not to spill solution on the equipment.

RED FLAG Make sure the patient isn't allergic to iodine solution; if he's allergic, use another antiseptic cleaning agent.

- Open the packet of water-soluble lubricant and apply it to the catheter tip.
- Attach the drainage bag to the other end of the catheter.
- If using a commercial kit, the drainage bag may be already attached.
- Make sure all tubing ends remain sterile; be sure the clamp at the emptying port of the drainage bag is closed to prevent urine leakage from the bag.
- Some drainage systems have an air-lock chamber to prevent bacteria from traveling to the bladder from urine in the drainage bag.

RED FLAG Some urologists and nurses use a syringe prefilled with water-soluble lubricant and instill the lubricant directly into the male urethra, instead of on the catheter tip. This method helps prevent trauma to the urethral lining and possible urinary tract infection (UTI). Check your facility's policy.

- Before inserting the catheter, inflate the balloon with sterile water to inspect for leaks.
- Attach the prefilled syringe to the Luer-Lok, then push the plunger and check for seepage as the balloon expands.
- Aspirate the solution to deflate the balloon.
- Inspect the catheter for resiliency. Rough, cracked catheters can injure the urethral mucosa during insertion, which can predispose the patient to infection.

For the female patient

■ Separate the labia majora and labia minora as widely as possible with the thumb, middle, and index fingers of your nondominant hand so you have a full view of the urinary meatus.

■ Keep the labia separated throughout the procedure so they don't obscure the urinary meatus or contaminate the area after it's cleaned.

■ Wipe one side of the urinary meatus with a sterile, cotton-tipped applicator (or pick up a sterile cotton ball with the plastic forceps) with a single downward motion.

■ Wipe the other side with another sterile applicator or cotton ball in the same way.

■ Wipe directly over the meatus with a third sterile applicator or cotton ball.

■ Take care not to contaminate your sterile glove.

For the male patient

■ Hold the penis with your nondominant hand.

■ If the patient is uncircumcised, retract the foreskin.

■ Lift and stretch the penis to a 60- to 90-degree angle.

■ Hold the penis this way throughout procedure to straighten the urethra and maintain a sterile field.

■ Use your dominant hand to clean the glans with a sterile cotton-tipped applicator or a sterile cotton ball held in forceps.

■ Clean in a circular motion, starting at the urinary meatus and working outward.

■ Repeat the procedure using another sterile applicator or cotton ball, taking care not to contaminate your sterile glove.

■ Pick up the catheter with your dominant hand and prepare to insert the lubricated tip into the urinary meatus.

■ To relax the sphincter, which facilitates insertion, ask the patient to cough as you insert the catheter. Tell him to breathe deeply and slowly to further relax the sphincter.

■ Hold the catheter close to its tip to ease insertion and control direction.

RED FLAG Never force a catheter during insertion. Maneuver it gently as the patient bears down or coughs. If you meet resistance, stop and notify physician. Sphincter spasms, strictures, misplacement in the vagina (in females), or an enlarged prostate (in males) may cause resistance.

Urinary catheter advancement

■ For the female patient, advance the catheter 2″ to 3″ (5 to
7.5 cm) while continuing to hold the labia apart (as shown) until
urine begins to flow.

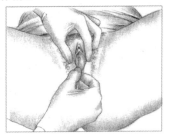

■ If the catheter is inadvertently inserted into the vagina, leave it
there as a landmark. Then begin the procedure over again using
new supplies.
■ For the male patient, advance the catheter to the bifurcation 5″ to
7½″ (12.5 to 19 cm) and check for urine flow (as shown).

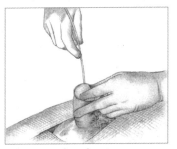

■ If the foreskin was retracted, replace it to prevent compromised
circulation and painful swelling.
■ When urine stops flowing, attach the pre-filled syringe to the
Luer-Lock.
■ Push the plunger and inflate the balloon to keep the catheter in
place in the bladder.

⚑ *RED FLAG Never inflate a balloon without establishing urine
flow, which assures that the catheter is in the bladder.*

■ Hang the collection bag below bladder level to prevent urine reflux into the bladder, which can cause infection, and to facilitate
gravity drainage of the bladder.

⚑ *RED FLAG Make sure that the tubing doesn't get tangled in the
bed rails.*

- Tape the catheter to the female patient's thigh to prevent possible tension on the urogenital trigone.
- Tape the catheter to the male patient's anterior thigh to prevent pressure on the urethra at the penoscrotal junction, which can lead to formation of urethrocutaneous fistulas.
- Securing the catheter with tape prevents traction on the bladder and alters the normal direction of urine flow in males.
- As an alternative, secure the catheter to the patient's thigh using a leg band with a Velcro closure.
- Using a thigh to secure the catheter decreases skin irritation, especially in patients with long-term indwelling catheters.
- Dispose of all used supplies properly.

SPECIAL CONSIDERATIONS

- A coude catheter may be indicated if the patient is a man older than 50 or has a history of previous surgery or prostate-related problems.

  RED FLAG When inserting a coude catheter, the curved tip should point upward.
- Several catheters are available with balloons of various sizes; each type has its own method of inflation and closure.
- Methods of balloon inflation and closure include the following:
  - Sterile solution or air may be injected through the inflation lumen; then, the end of the injection port is folded over itself and fastened with a clamp or rubber band.
  - The catheter may be inflated when a seal in the end of the inflation lumen is penetrated with a needle or the tip of the solution-filled syringe.
  - The catheter may be self-inflatable when a propositioned clamp is loosened.
- Injecting a balloon with air makes identifying leaks difficult and doesn't guarantee deflation of the balloon for removal.
- The balloon size determines the amount of solution needed for inflation; the exact amount is usually printed on the distal end of the catheter port used for inflating the balloon.
- If the physician orders a urine specimen, obtain it from the urine receptacle with a specimen collection container at the time of catheterization and send it to the laboratory with an appropriate laboratory request form.
- Connect the drainage bag when urine stops flowing.
- Inspect the catheter and tubing periodically to detect compression or kinking that could obstruct urine flow.

- Reinforce the explanation regarding gravity drainage so the patient realizes the importance of keeping the drainage tubing and collection bag lower than the bladder at all times.
- If necessary, provide the patient with detailed instructions for performing clean intermittent self-catheterization.
- For monitoring purposes, empty the collection bag at least every 8 hours.
- Excessive fluid volume may require more frequent emptying to prevent injury to the urethra and bladder wall and traction on the catheter, which may cause discomfort.

RED FLAG Observe the patient carefully for adverse reactions caused by removing excessive volumes of residual urine, such as hypovolemic shock.

RED FLAG Check facility policy to determine maximum amount of urine that may be drained at one time (some facilities limit the amount to 700 to 1,000 ml). Clamp the catheter at the first sign of adverse reaction, and notify the physician.

- Some hospitals encourage changing catheters at regular intervals, such as every 30 days, if the patient has long-term continuous drainage.
- If the patient will be discharged with a long-term indwelling catheter, reinforce teaching with him and his family about aspects of daily catheter maintenance, including:
  - care of skin and urinary meatus
  - signs and symptoms of UTI or obstruction
  - how to irrigate catheter (if appropriate)
  - how to use a leg bag during the day or while out and a larger drainage bag at night or when at home, as appropriate
  - importance of adequate fluid intake to maintain patency
  - need for a home care nurse to visit every 4 to 6 weeks, or as needed, to change catheter.

COMPLICATIONS

Complications include a UTI, which can result from introduction of bacteria into the bladder. Improper catheter insertion can cause traumatic injury to urethral and bladder mucosa. Bladder atony or spasms can result from rapid decompression of a severely distended bladder.

DOCUMENTATION

- Record the date, time, size, and type of indwelling catheter used and the volume of fluid or air used to inflate the balloon.

Urinary diversion techniques

A cystostomy or a nephrostomy can be used to create a temporary or permanent urinary diversion, to relieve obstruction from an inoperable tumor, or provide an outlet for urine after cystectomy.

A temporary diversion can relieve obstruction from a calculus or ureteral edema.

In a cystostomy, a catheter is inserted percutaneously through the suprapubic area into the bladder. In a nephrostomy, a catheter is inserted percutaneously through the flank into the renal pelvis.

CYSTOSTOMY **NEPHROSTOMY**

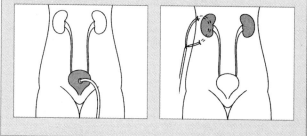

- Describe the amount, color, and other characteristics of urine emptied from bladder. (Your facility may require an intake and output sheet for fluid-balance data.)
- If large volumes of urine have been emptied, describe the patient's tolerance of the procedure.
- Note whether a urine specimen was sent for laboratory analysis.

Nephrostomy and cystostomy tube care

Urinary diversion techniques ensure adequate drainage from the kidneys or bladder and help prevent urinary tract infection or kidney failure. (See *Urinary diversion techniques*.)

A nephrostomy tube drains urine directly from a kidney when a disorder (such as calculi in the ureter or ureteropelvic junction or an obstructing tumor) inhibits normal urine flow. The tubes are usually placed percutaneously; sometimes they're surgically inserted. Draining urine with a nephrostomy tube allows kidney tissue damaged by obstructive disease to heal. A cystostomy tube drains urine from the bladder, diverting it from the urethra. The tubes are used after certain gynecologic procedures, bladder surgery, prostatectomy, and for severe urethral strictures or traumatic injury. They're inserted about 2″ (5 cm) above the symphysis pubis; a cystostomy tube may be used alone or with an indwelling urethral catheter.

CONTRAINDICATIONS
None known.

EQUIPMENT
For dressing changes
4″ × 4″ gauze pads ● povidone-iodine solution or povidone-iodine pads ● sterile cup or emesis basin ● paper bag ● linen-saver pad ● clean gloves (for dressing removal) ● sterile gloves (for new dressing) ● precut 4″ × 4″ drain dressings or transparent semipermeable dressings ● adhesive tape (preferably hypoallergenic)

For nephrostomy-tube irrigation
3-ml syringe ● alcohol pad or povidone-iodine pad ● normal saline solution ● hemostat (optional)

Preparation of equipment
■ Check with the patient and his chart to determine if he is allergic to iodine or shellfish.
■ Wash your hands.
■ Assemble the equipment at the patient's bedside.
■ Open several packages of gauze pads, place them in the sterile cup or emesis basin, and pour the povidone-iodine solution over them.
■ Open a commercially packaged kit (if available), using sterile technique.
■ Fill the cup with antiseptic solution.
■ Open the paper bag and place it away from the other equipment to avoid contaminating the sterile field.

ESSENTIAL STEPS
■ Verify the patient's identity using two patient identifiers, such as the patient's name and identification number.
■ Wash your hands, provide privacy, and reinforce the explanation of the procedure to the patient.

Changing a dressing
■ Put the patient on his back (for a cystostomy tube) or the side opposite the tube (for a nephrostomy tube).

- Place the linen-saver pad under the patient to absorb drainage.
- Put on clean gloves.
- Carefully remove the tape around the tube.
- Remove wet or soiled dressings.
- Discard the tape and dressing in the paper bag.
- Remove the gloves and discard them in the bag.
- Wash your hands.
- Put on sterile gloves.
- Pick up a saturated pad or dip a dry one into the cup of antiseptic solution.
- To clean the wound, wipe only once with each pad or sponge, moving from the insertion site outward.
- Discard the used pad or sponge in the paper bag.
- To avoid contaminating your gloves, don't touch the bag.
- Pick up a sterile 4″ × 4″ drain dressing and place it around the tube.
- If necessary, overlap two drain dressings to provide maximum absorption. Alternatively, depending on your facility's policy, apply a transparent semipermeable dressing over the site and tubing to allow observation of the site.
- Secure the dressing with hypoallergenic tape.
- Tape the tube to the patient's lateral abdomen to prevent tension.
- Dispose of all equipment appropriately.
- Clean the patient as necessary.

Irrigating a nephrostomy tube

- Confirm the physician's order.
- Fill the 3-ml syringe with the normal saline solution.
- Clean the junction of the nephrostomy tube and drainage tube with the alcohol pad or povidone-iodine pad, and disconnect the tubes. A stopcock may be used to prevent unnecessary pulling of the nephrostomy tube and to establish a stable, clean access port.
- Insert the syringe into the nephrostomy tube opening, and instill 2 to 3 ml of normal saline solution into the tube.

RED FLAG Never irrigate a nephrostomy tube with more than 5 ml of solution because the capacity of the renal pelvis is usually 4 to 8 ml. (The purpose of irrigation is to keep the tube patent, not to lavage the renal pelvis.)

- Slowly aspirate the solution back into the syringe.

RED FLAG Never pull back on the plunger. If the solution doesn't return, remove the syringe from the tube and reattach it to the drainage tubing to allow the solution to drain by gravity.

- Dispose of all equipment appropriately.

SPECIAL CONSIDERATIONS
- Change dressings once per day or more often as needed.
- Irrigate a cystostomy tube as you would an indwelling urinary catheter.
- Perform irrigation to avoid damaging any suture lines.
- Curve a cystostomy tube to prevent kinks; kinks are likely if the patient lies on the insertion site.
- Check a nephrostomy tube frequently for kinks or obstructions.
- Suspect an obstruction when the amount of urine in the drainage bag decreases or the amount of urine around the insertion site increases.
- If a blood clot or mucus plug obstructs a nephrostomy or cystostomy tube, try milking the tube to restore its patency.
- Check a cystostomy hourly for postoperative urologic patients.
- To check tube patency, note the amount of urine in the drainage bag and check the patient's bladder for distention.
- Keep the drainage bag below the level of the kidney at all times.
- Notify the physician immediately if the tube becomes dislodged.
- Cover the site with a sterile dressing.
- While clamping the nephrostomy tube, monitor the patient for flank pain and fever, and monitor urine output.
- Reinforce the explanation of how to clean the insertion site with soap and water, check for skin breakdown, and change dressing daily.
- Reinforce how to change and how and when to wash the leg bag or drainage bag.
- Remind the patient to increase fluid intake to 3 qt (3 L) daily, if not contraindicated.
- Reinforce signs of infection (red skin; white, yellow, or green drainage; or pain at the insertion site and fever) and tell the patient to report them to his physician.

COMPLICATIONS
Introduction of bacteria in the urinary tract can cause urinary tract infection.

DOCUMENTATION
- Record the color and amount of drainage.
- Note the amount and type of irrigant used.
- Document whether you obtained a complete return.
- Document a description of the insertion site and any drainage from the site.

Papanicolaou test assistance

A Papanicolaou test, also known as a *Pap test* or *Pap smear*, is a cytologic test for early detection of cervical cancer. The test involves scraping secretions from the cervix, spreading them on a slide, and coating the slide with fixative spray or solution to preserve specimen cells for nuclear staining. Cytologic evaluation reveals cell maturity, morphology, and metabolic activity. A Pap test also permits cytologic evaluation of the vaginal pool, prostatic secretions, urine, gastric secretions, cavity fluids, bronchial aspirations, and sputum. The ThinPrep Pap test is a tool for early detection of cervical cancer. (See *ThinPrep Pap test.*)

CONTRAINDICATIONS
None known.

EQUIPMENT
Bivalve vaginal speculum ● gloves ● Pap stick (wooden spatula) ● long cotton-tipped applicator ● three glass microscope slides ● fixative (a commercial spray or 95% ethyl alcohol solution) ● adjustable lamp ● drape ● laboratory request forms

PREPARATION OF EQUIPMENT
■ Select a speculum of appropriate size.
■ Gather the equipment in the examining room.
■ Label the glass slides with the patient's name and "E," "C," and "V" to differentiate endocervical, cervical, and vaginal specimens.

ThinPrep Pap test

Since 1996, the ThinPrep Pap test has been used as a replacement for the conventional Pap test for cervical cancer screening.

Most laboratories in the United States can process this test, which is significantly more effective than traditional tests for detecting cervical abnormalities in many patient populations.

The ThinPrep Pap test can also be used to test for human papillomavirus, a sexually transmitted disease linked to cervical cancer, and to diagnose *Chlamydia trachomatis* and *Neisseria gonorrhoeae.*

ESSENTIAL STEPS

■ Verify the patient's identity using two patient identifiers, such as the patient's name and identification number.
■ Reinforce the explanation of the procedure to the patient.
■ Wash your hands.
■ Instruct the patient to void before the examination.
■ Provide privacy.
■ Instruct the patient to undress below the waist.
■ Instruct her to sit on the examination table and drape her genital region.
■ Place the patient in the lithotomy position, with her feet in the stirrups and her buttocks extended slightly beyond the edge of the table.
■ Adjust the drape.
■ Adjust the lamp so that it fully illuminates the genital area.
■ Fold back the corner of the drape to expose the perineum.
■ Put on gloves.
■ Assist the physician or nurse to take the speculum in his dominant hand and moisten it with warm water to ease insertion.

RED FLAG Avoid using water-soluble lubricants, which interfere with accurate laboratory testing.

■ Avoid using water-soluble lubricants, which interfere with accurate laboratory testing.
■ Warn the patient that she's about to be touched to avoid startling her.
■ The labia will be gently separated by the examiner with the thumb and forefinger of his nondominant hand.
■ Encourage the patient to take several deep breaths.
■ The speculum will be inserted into the vagina.
■ When it's in place, the blades will be opened slowly to expose the cervix.
■ The blades will be locked in place.
■ A cotton-tipped applicator will be inserted through the speculum $\frac{1}{5}$" into the cervical os.
■ The applicator will be rotated 360 degrees to obtain an endocervical specimen.
■ The applicator will be removed and gently rolled in a circle across the slide marked "E."
■ To prevent cell destruction, the applicator shouldn't be rubbed on the slide.
■ ___mediately place the slide in a fixative solution or spray it with ___ative to prevent drying of cells.
___mall curved end of the Pap stick will be inserted through ___culum and placed directly over the cervical os.

- The stick will be gently but firmly rotated to scrape cells loose.
- The stick will be removed, and the specimen spread across the slide marked "C," and fixed immediately, as before.
- The opposite end of the Pap stick or a cotton-tipped applicator will be inserted through the speculum, and the posterior fornix or vaginal pool will be scraped. This area collects cells from the endometrium, vagina, and cervix.
- The stick or applicator will be removed, the specimen will be spread across the slide marked "V," and fixed immediately.
- The speculum will be unlocked (to ease removal and avoid accidentally pinching the vaginal wall) and then withdrawn.
- A bimanual exam will be performed.
- Remove and discard gloves.
- Remove the patient's feet from the stirrups and help her to a sitting position.
- Provide privacy for her to dress and towels that she can use to clean herself.
- Fill out the appropriate laboratory request forms, including the date of the patient's last menses.

SPECIAL CONSIDERATIONS

- Many preventable factors can interfere with the Pap test's accuracy.
- Remind the patient to avoid vaginal douching, administering vaginal medications, and sexual intercourse 48 hours before specimen collection.
- Schedule the test 5 to 6 days before menses or 1 week after.
- Application of topical antibiotics promotes rapid, heavy shedding of cells and requires postponement of the Pap test for at least 1 month.
- If the patient has had a complete hysterectomy, collect test specimens from the vaginal pool and cuff.
- Reinforce the explanation of the procedure and answer any questions to lessen the patient's anxiety.

COMPLICATIONS

Failure to unlock speculum blades before removal can pinch vaginal tissue. Rough handling of the speculum can cause severe cramping. Scraping an inflamed cervix with the Pap stick can cause bleeding.

DOCUMENTATION

- Record the date and time of specimen collection.

9

INTEGUMENTARY CARE

Besides influencing a person's self-image, the skin performs many physiologic functions. It protects internal body structures from the environment and from potential pathogens; it regulates body temperature and homeostasis; and it serves as an organ of sensation and excretion. When skin integrity is compromised by pressure ulcers, burns, or other lesions, nursing care focuses on taking steps to prevent or control infection, promote new skin growth, control pain, and provide emotional support.

Closed-wound drain management

A closed-wound drain promotes healing and prevents swelling by suctioning serosanguineous fluid that accumulates at a wound site. It's typically inserted during surgery when substantial postoperative drainage is anticipated. By removing postoperative fluid, it reduces the risk of infection and skin breakdown and the frequency of dressing changes. The system consists of perforated tubing connected to a portable vacuum unit. The distal end of the tubing lies inside the wound and usually exits the body from a puncture site other than the primary suture line, to preserve integrity of the surgical wound. The drain is usually sutured to the skin, and the tubing exit site is treated as an additional surgical wound. If the wound produces heavy drainage, the closed-wound drain may be left in place for a longer time. Drainage must be emptied and measured frequently to maintain maximum suction and prevent strain on the suture line. Hemovac and Jackson-Pratt closed drainage systems are commonly used.

CONTRAINDICATIONS
None known.

EQUIPMENT

Graduated biohazard cylinder ● sterile laboratory container, if needed ● alcohol pads ● gloves ● gown ● face shield ● trash bag ● sterile gauze pads ● antiseptic cleaning agent ● prepackaged povidone-iodine swabs ● label (optional)

ESSENTIAL STEPS

- Reinforce the explanation of the procedure to the patient and provide privacy.
- Identify allergies, especially to povidone-iodine or other topical antiseptics.
- Wash your hands and put on gloves and face shield or goggles.
- Unclip the vacuum unit from the patient's bed or gown.
- Using sterile technique, release the vacuum by removing the spout plug on the collection chamber.
- The container expands completely as it draws in air.
- Empty the unit's contents into a graduated biohazard cylinder, and note the amount, appearance, consistency, and odor of the drainage.
- If diagnostic tests will be performed on the specimen, pour the drainage directly into a sterile laboratory container, note the amount, label the specimen, and send it to the laboratory.
- Clean the unit's spout and plug with an alcohol pad using sterile technique.
- To reestablish the vacuum that creates the drain's suction power, fully compress the vacuum unit.
- Compress the unit with one hand to maintain the vacuum and replace the spout plug. (See *Using a closed-wound drainage system,* page 250.)
- Check the patency of the equipment.
- Make sure the tubing is free from twists, kinks, and leaks; the drainage system must be airtight to work properly.
- The vacuum unit should remain compressed when you release manual pressure.
- If rapid reinflation occurs, indicating an air leak, recompress the unit and resecure the spout plug.
- Fasten the vacuum unit to the patient's gown below wound level to promote drainage.
- To prevent dislodgment, don't apply tension on drainage tubing when fastening the unit.
- Remove and discard your gloves and wash your hands.
- Check the sutures that secure the drain to the patient's skin.
- Monitor for signs of pulling or tearing and swelling or infection.

Using a closed-wound drainage system

This system draws drainage from a wound site, such as the chest wall postmastectomy shown at left, by means of straight or Y-tubing. To empty the drainage, remove the plug and empty into a graduated cylinder. To reestablish suction, compress the drainage unit against a firm surface to expel air and, while holding it down, replace the plug, as shown. The same principle is used for the Jackson-Pratt bulb drain, shown below right.

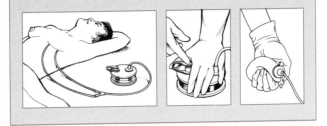

- Put on gloves and gently clean the sutures with sterile gauze pads soaked in an antiseptic cleaning agent or with a povidone-iodine swab.
- Properly dispose of drainage, solutions, and trash bag, and clean or dispose of soiled equipment and supplies according to facility policy.

SPECIAL CONSIDERATIONS

- Empty the drain and measure its contents once during each shift, more often if drainage is excessive or if the physician orders.

  ⚑ *RED FLAG Notify the supervising RN and physician immediately if the amount of drainage is excessive per his orders or if drainage consists of bright red blood.*

- Removing excess drainage maintains maximum suction and avoids straining the drain's suture line.
- Empty and measure the drainage before the patient ambulates to prevent the weight of drainage from pulling on the drain.

  ⚑ *RED FLAG Be careful not to mistake chest tubes for closed-wound drains because the vacuum of a chest tube should never be released.*

- If the patient is to be discharged to home with a drain in place, reinforce teaching related to emptying and measuring the drainage and caring for the drain site.

COMPLICATIONS

Occlusion of tubing by fibrin, clots, or other particles can reduce or obstruct drainage. An infection can occur at the drain site or the drainage can become infected.

DOCUMENTATION

- Record the date and time you empty the drain.
- Describe the appearance of the drain site.
- Note the presence of swelling or signs of infection.
- Note the patient's tolerance of treatment.
- Record the color, consistency, type, and odor of the drainage.
- Document the amount of the drainage on the input and output sheet.
- If there's more than one closed-wound drain, number the drains and record the above information separately for each drainage site.

Pressure ulcer care

Treatment and care of pressure ulcers involves relieving pressure, restoring circulation, promoting adequate nutrition, and resolving or managing related disorders. Care may require special pressure-reducing devices, such as beds, mattresses, mattress overlays, and chair cushions. Other measures include decreasing risk factors, use of topical treatments, wound cleaning, debridement, and use of dressings to support moist wound healing. Use standard precaution guidelines of the Centers for Disease Control and Prevention when giving care. The specific treatment techniques employed and the effectiveness and duration of treatment depend on the characteristics of the pressure ulcer and the stage of the ulcer. (See *Staging pressure ulcers,* page 252.)

CONTRAINDICATIONS

None known.

EQUIPMENT

Hypoallergenic tape or elastic netting ● overbed table ● piston-type irrigating system ● two pairs of gloves ● normal saline solution ● sterile 4″ × 4″ gauze pads ● sterile cotton swabs ● selected topical dressing ● linen-saver pads ● impervious plastic trash bag ● disposable wound-measuring device

Staging pressure ulcers

You can use pressure ulcer characteristics gained from your observations to stage the pressure ulcer, as described here. Staging reflects the anatomic depth of exposed tissue. Keep in mind that if the wound contains necrotic tissue, you won't be able to determine the stage until you can see the wound base.

STAGE I
- In light-colored skin, a defined persistently red area
- In darker skin, a defined persistently red, blue, or purple area

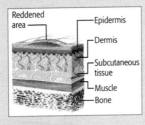

Reddened area — Epidermis
— Dermis
— Subcutaneous tissue
— Muscle
— Bone

STAGE II
- Partial-thickness skin loss of epidermis or dermis
- Superficial ulcer
- Abrasion, blister, or shallow crater

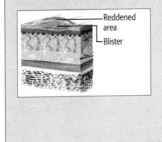

— Reddened area
— Blister

STAGE III
- Full-thickness skin loss
- Damage or necrosis of subcutaneous tissue
- May extend down to but not through fascia
- Deep crater with or without undermining of adjacent tissue

STAGE IV
- Full-thickness skin loss
- Extensive destruction, tissue necrosis, or damage to muscle, bone, or support structures
- Possible tunneling and sinus tracts

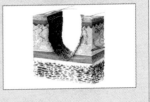

PREPARATION OF EQUIPMENT
- Assemble the equipment at the patient's bedside.
- Cut the tape into strips.
- Loosen lids on cleaning solutions and drugs.

■ Loosen existing dressing edges and tapes.
■ Attach an impervious plastic trash bag to the overbed table.

ESSENTIAL STEPS
Cleaning the pressure ulcer
■ Provide privacy and reinforce the explanation of the procedure to allay fear and promote cooperation.
■ Verify the patent's identity using two patient identifiers, such as the patient's name and identification number.
■ Wash your hands.
■ Position the patient for comfort and easy access to the site.
■ Cover bed linens with a linen-saver pad to prevent soiling.
■ Open the normal saline solution container and the piston syringe.
■ Pour solution carefully into a clean or sterile irrigation container.
■ Put the piston syringe into the opening of the irrigation container.
■ Open the packages of supplies.
■ Put on gloves before removing the old dressing and exposing the pressure ulcer.
■ Note any drainage on the soiled dressing and discard it in the impervious plastic trash bag.
■ Inspect the wound. Note the color, amount, and odor of any drainage or necrotic debris.
■ Measure the wound perimeter with a disposable wound-measuring device.
■ Apply full force of the piston syringe to irrigate the ulcer, remove necrotic debris, and decrease bacteria in the wound.
■ For nonnecrotic wounds, use less pressure to prevent damage.
■ Remove and discard your soiled gloves, wash your hands, and put on a fresh pair of gloves.
■ Insert a sterile cotton swab into the wound to monitor for tunneling or undermining.
■ Monitor and note the condition of the clean wound and surrounding skin.
■ Notify the supervising RN or wound care specialist if adherent necrotic material is present.
■ Apply the topical dressing.

Applying a moist saline gauze dressing
■ Irrigate the ulcer with normal saline solution. Blot surrounding skin dry.
■ Moisten the gauze dressing with normal saline solution.
■ Gently place the dressing over the surface of the ulcer.

- To separate surfaces within the wound, gently place a dressing between opposing wound surfaces. Don't pack the gauze tightly. Apply a dry, external dressing and secure with tape.
- Change the dressing often enough to keep the wound moist.

Applying a hydrocolloid dressing

- Irrigate the ulcer with normal saline solution. Blot surrounding skin dry.
- Choose a clean, dry, presized dressing, or cut one to overlap the pressure ulcer by about 1" (2.5 cm).
- Remove the dressing from its package, remove the release paper, and apply the dressing to the wound. Carefully smooth wrinkles and air pockets as you apply the dressing.
- If using tape to secure the dressing, apply a skin sealant to the intact skin around the ulcer.
- When dry, tape the dressing to the skin. Avoid tension or pressure.
- Remove and discard your gloves and other refuse.
- Wash your hands.
- Change a hydrocolloid dressing every 2 to 7 days or when soiled.
- Discontinue if signs of infection are present.

Applying a transparent dressing

- Irrigate the ulcer with normal saline solution. Blot surrounding skin dry.
- Clean and dry the wound as described above.
- Select a dressing to overlap the ulcer by 2" (5.1 cm).
- Gently lay the dressing over the ulcer. Don't stretch it.
- Press firmly on the edges of the dressing to promote adherence.
- Tape edges to prevent them from curling.
- Clean the site with an alcohol pad and cover it with a transparent dressing.
- Change the dressing every 3 to 7 days or when soiled, depending on drainage.

Applying an alginate dressing

- Irrigate the ulcer with normal saline solution. Blot surrounding skin dry.
- Apply the alginate dressing to the ulcer surface. Cover with a second dressing (such as gauze pads). Secure with tape or elastic netting.
- If drainage is heavy, change the dressing once or twice daily for the first 3 to 5 days.

■ As drainage decreases, change the dressing less frequently—every 2 to 4 days or as ordered.
■ When drainage stops or the wound bed is dry, notify the supervising RN and physician, who will order an alternative treatment.

Applying a foam dressing
■ Irrigate the ulcer with normal saline solution. Blot surrounding skin dry.
■ Lay the foam dressing over the ulcer.
■ Use tape, elastic netting, or gauze to hold the dressing in place.
■ Change the dressing when the foam no longer absorbs the exudate.

Applying a hydrogel dressing
■ Irrigate the ulcer with normal saline solution. Blot surrounding skin dry.
■ Apply gel to the wound bed.
■ Cover the area with a second dressing.
■ Change the dressing as needed, to keep the wound bed moist.
■ If you choose a sheet form dressing, cut it to match the wound base.
■ Hydrogel dressings also come in a prepackaged, saturated gauze to fill "dead space." Follow the manufacturer's directions.

Preventing pressure ulcers
■ Turn and reposition the patient every 1 to 2 hours unless contraindicated.
■ Use an air, gel, or 4″ foam mattress for those who can't turn themselves or those who are turned on a schedule.
■ Low- or high-air-loss therapy may be indicated.
■ Implement active or passive range-of-motion exercises.
■ To save time, combine exercises with bathing if applicable.
■ Lift rather than slide the patient when turning to prevent shearing forces.
■ Use a turning sheet and get help from coworkers.
■ Use pillows to position the patient and increase his comfort.
■ Eliminate sheet wrinkles.
■ Post a turning schedule at his bedside.
■ Avoid the trochanter position. Instead, position at a 30-degree angle.
■ Avoid raising the bed more than 30 degrees for long periods.
■ Adjust or pad appliances, casts, or splints, to ensure proper fit.
■ Gently apply lotion after bathing to keep skin moist.

■ Clean and dry soiled skin. Apply a protective moisture barrier.
■ Ensure adequate nutritional intake and hydration.

SPECIAL CONSIDERATIONS

■ Prevention helps avoid extensive therapy and increased costs of hospitalization; measures include ensuring adequate nourishment and mobility to relieve pressure and promote circulation.
■ Direct the patient in a chair or wheelchair to shift his weight every 15 minutes. Limit sitting to 1 hour at a time.
■ An over-the-bed trapeze may enable the patient to change position in bed and shift his weight more easily.
■ Instruct a paraplegic patient to shift his weight by doing push-ups.
■ Tell the patient to avoid heat lamps and harsh soaps.
■ Avoid using elbow and heel protectors with a single narrow strap.
■ Avoid using artificial sheepskin. It doesn't reduce pressure.
■ Repair of stages 3 and 4 ulcers may require surgical intervention.
■ Reinforce with the patient and his family the importance of prevention, position changes, and treatment. Remind them of the proper methods and encourage participation.
■ Reinforce that the patient should follow a diet with adequate calories, protein, vitamins, and hydration.
■ Reinforce that the patient should notify the physician at the first signs or symptoms of skin breakdown to obtain treatment instructions.
■ Reinforce signs and symptoms of infection and when to notify the physician.

COMPLICATIONS

Infection produces foul-smelling drainage, persistent pain, severe erythema, induration, and elevated skin and body temperatures. Infection may lead to cellulitis and septicemia.

DOCUMENTATION

■ Record the date and time of initial and subsequent treatments.
■ Detail preventive measures performed.
■ Note the ulcer's location, size (length, width, depth), color, and appearance.
■ Record the drainage's amount, odor, color, and consistency.
■ Document the surrounding skin's condition and temperature.
■ Record body temperature daily.
■ Monitor the pressure ulcers at least weekly and update the plan.
■ Record physician notification.

■ Document the amount of time spent out of bed in the chair or ambulating and the turning and positioning schedule.

Suture removal

The goal of suture removal is to remove sutures from a healed wound without damaging newly formed tissue. Timing depends on the shape, size, and location of the sutured incision; the absence of inflammation, drainage, and infection; and the patient's general condition. If the wound is sufficiently healed, sutures are removed 7 to 10 days after insertion. Techniques for removal depend on the method of suturing. Sterile procedures are required. Sutures are usually removed by a physician or qualified nurse.

CONTRAINDICATIONS
■ Insufficient wound healing

EQUIPMENT
Waterproof trash bag ● adjustable light ● clean gloves, if the wound is dressed ● sterile forceps or sterile hemostat ● normal saline solution ● sterile gauze pads ● antiseptic cleaning agent ● sterile curve-tipped suture scissors ● povidone-iodine pads ● adhesive butterfly strips or adhesive strips and compound benzoin tincture or other skin protectant (optional)

Prepackaged, sterile suture-removal trays are available.

PREPARATION OF EQUIPMENT
■ Assemble the equipment in the patient's room.
■ Check the expiration date on each sterile package and inspect for tears.
■ Open the waterproof trash bag, and place it near the patient's bed.
■ Turn down the top of the trash bag to provide a wide opening and prevent contamination of instruments or gloves by touching the bag's edge.

ESSENTIAL STEPS
■ Verify the patent's identity using two patient identifiers, such as the patient's name and identification number.
■ Check patient allergies, especially to adhesive tape, povidone-iodine or other topical solutions or drugs.
■ Reinforce the explanation of the procedure to the patient.

■ Remind the patient that the procedure is usually painless, but he may feel a tickling sensation, and that removing stitches won't weaken the incision.

■ Provide privacy.

■ Position the patient so he's comfortable without placing undue tension on the suture line.

■ To avoid nausea or dizziness, have the patient recline.

■ Adjust the light so it shines directly on the suture line.

■ Wash your hands.

■ Put on clean gloves to remove the dressing, if present.

■ Discard the dressing and gloves in the waterproof trash bag.

■ Monitor the wound for gaping, drainage, inflammation, signs of infection, or embedded sutures.

■ Notify the supervising RN and physician if the wound has failed to heal properly.

RED FLAG Absence of a healing ridge under the suture line 5 to 7 days after the incision indicates that continued support and protection are needed.

■ The physician or qualified nurse performing the procedure will put on sterile gloves.

■ Help him establish a sterile work area with needed equipment and supplies.

■ Put on sterile gloves.

■ Open the sterile suture removal tray if he's using one.

■ Using sterile technique, help him clean the suture line, which moistens the sutures to ease removal.

■ Soften them further, if needed, with normal saline solution.

■ The physician or qualified nurse will proceed according to the type of suture he's removing.

■ The visible part of a suture is contaminated; the physician or qualified nurse will cut the sutures at the skin surface on one side and lift and pull the visible end off the skin.

■ He may start by removing every other suture to maintain support for the incision, and then remove the remaining sutures.

■ After suture removal, wipe the incision with gauze pads soaked in an antiseptic cleaning agent or with a povidone-iodine pad.

■ Apply a light sterile gauze dressing if needed.

■ Discard your gloves.

■ Make sure the patient is comfortable.

■ After checking the physician's orders, inform the patient when he may shower, usually in 1 or 2 days if the incision is dry and heals well.

■ Properly dispose of the solutions and trash bag. Clean or dispose of soiled equipment and supplies.

SPECIAL CONSIDERATIONS

■ A typical guideline follows for suture removal, but the physician's orders may vary:
  - head and neck—3 to 5 days after insertion
  - chest and abdomen—5 to 7 days after insertion
  - lower extremities—7 to 10 days after insertion.
■ For interrupted sutures or an incompletely healed suture line, the physician may not remove all of the sutures; some sutures may be left in place for 1 to 2 days to support the suture line.
■ If both retention and regular sutures are in place, confer with the physician to determine the removal sequence so it can be communicated to the patient.
■ Retention sutures usually remain in place for 14 to 21 days.
■ Retention sutures give added support to obese or slow-healing patients.
■ Carefully clean the suture line before mattress sutures are removed to decrease the risk of infection when the visible, contaminated part of the stitch is too small to cut twice for sterile removal and must be pulled through the tissue.
■ After mattress sutures are removed, monitor the suture line for subsequent infection.
■ If the wound dehisces during or after suture removal, apply butterfly adhesive strips or adhesive strips to support and approximate the edges and help the physician repair the wound.
■ Apply butterfly adhesive strips or adhesive strips after suture removal for added support of the incision line and prevention of wide scar formation.
■ Use skin protectant to ensure adherence.
■ Leave the strips in place for 3 to 5 days or until they fall off.
■ Before discharge, reinforce with the patient how to remove the dressing and care for the wound.
■ Reinforce that he should call the physician immediately if he observes wound discharge or other abnormal changes.
■ Remind the patient that the redness surrounding the incision should gradually disappear with only a thin line remaining after a few weeks.

COMPLICATIONS

Complications include dehiscence of the suture line and infection.

DOCUMENTATION

■ Record the date and time of suture removal.
■ Note the type and number of sutures and the appearance of the suture line.

■ Record signs of wound complications.
■ Note dressings or adhesive strips applied.
■ Document the patient's tolerance of the procedure.

Unna's boot

Unna's boot is a commercially prepared, medicated gauze compression dressing that wraps around the foot and leg. It can be used to treat uninfected, nonnecrotic leg and foot ulcers caused by venous insufficiency and stasis dermatitis. Alternatively, Unna's paste (gelatin, zinc oxide, calamine lotion, and glycerin) may be applied to the ulcer and covered with lightweight gauze. Effectiveness results from compression (bandage) and moisture (paste).

CONTRAINDICATIONS
■ Allergy to any ingredient used in the paste
■ Arterial ulcers
■ Weeping eczema
■ Cellulitis

EQUIPMENT
Scrub sponge with ordered cleaning agent ● normal saline solution ● commercially prepared gauze bandage saturated with Unna's paste (or Unna's paste and lightweight gauze) ● bandage scissors ● gloves ● elastic bandage to cover Unna's boot ● extra gauze for excessive drainage (optional)

ESSENTIAL STEPS
■ Verify the patent's identity using two patient identifiers, such as the patient's name and identification number.
■ Reinforce the explanation of the procedure and provide privacy.
■ Wash your hands and put on gloves.
■ Monitor the ulcer's size, drainage, and appearance and the surrounding skin. Monitor the neurovascular status of the affected foot to ensure adequate circulation.

RED FLAG If you don't detect a pulse in the foot, check with the supervising RN and physician before applying Unna's boot.

■ Clean the affected area with the sponge and cleaning agent to retard bacterial growth and remove dirt and wound debris, which may create pressure points after you apply the bandage. Rinse with normal saline solution.
■ If a commercially prepared gauze bandage isn't ordered, spread Unna's paste evenly on the leg and foot; cover with the lightweight gauze.

■ Apply three to four layers of paste interspersed with layers of gauze.

■ Apply gauze or the prepared bandage in a spiral motion, from just above the toes to the knee. (See *How to wrap Unna's boot,* page 262.)

■ Cover the heel; the wrap should be snug but not tight. To cover the area completely, make sure each turn overlaps the previous one by one-half of the bandage width.

■ Continue wrapping the patient's leg up to the knee, using firm, even pressure.

■ Stop the dressing 1″ (2.5 cm) below the popliteal fossa to prevent irritation when the knee is bent.

■ Mold the boot with your free hand as you apply the bandage to make it smooth and even.

■ Cover the boot with an elastic bandage to provide compression.

■ Instruct the patient to remain in bed with his leg outstretched and elevated on a pillow until the paste dries (about 30 minutes).

RED FLAG Monitor the patient's foot for signs of impairment, such as cyanosis, loss of feeling, and swelling, which indicate the bandage is too tight and must be removed.

■ Leave the boot on for 5 to 7 days or as ordered.

■ Change the boot weekly or as ordered to monitor the underlying skin and ulcer healing. Remove the boot by unwrapping the bandage from the knee back to the foot.

SPECIAL CONSIDERATIONS

■ If the boot is applied over a swollen leg, it must be changed as the edema subsides—if necessary, more frequently than every 5 days.

■ Don't make reverse turns while wrapping the bandage. This can create excessive pressure areas that may cause discomfort as the bandage hardens.

■ Reinforce the explanation of the procedure to the patient.

■ Remind the patient to walk on and handle the wrap carefully to avoid damaging it.

■ Remind the patient that the boot will stiffen but won't be as hard as a cast.

■ Remind the patient that before bathing, he should cover the boot with a plastic kitchen trash bag sealed at the knee with an elastic bandage to avoid getting the boot wet. A wet boot softens and loses it effectiveness.

■ Reinforce that he should take a sponge bath if his safety is a concern.

How to wrap Unna's boot

After cleaning the skin thoroughly, flex the patient's knee. Starting with his foot positioned at a right angle to his leg, wrap the medicated gauze bandage firmly—not tightly—around his foot. Make sure the dressing covers his heel. Continue wrapping upward, overlapping the dressing slightly with each turn. Smooth the boot with your free hand as you go, as shown below.

Stop wrapping about 1" (2.5 cm) below the knee. If necessary, make a 2" (5.1-cm) slit in the boot just below the knee to relieve constriction that may develop as the dressing hardens.

If drainage is excessive, wrap a roller gauze dressing over the Unna's boot. As the final layer, wrap an elastic bandage in a figure-eight pattern.

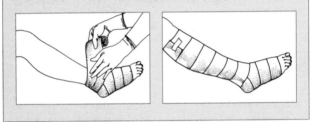

COMPLICATIONS
Contact dermatitis can occur from application of Unna's boot.

DOCUMENTATION
- Record the date and time of application and presence of a pulse in the affected foot.
- Specify which leg was bandaged; describe skin appearance before and after application.
- Record the equipment used (a commercially prepared bandage or Unna's paste and lightweight gauze).
- Note an allergic reaction.

Vacuum-assisted closure pressure therapy assistance

Vacuum-assisted closure (VAC) pressure therapy (also known as *negative pressure wound therapy*) is used to enhance delayed or impaired wound healing. The device applies localized subatmospheric pressure to draw the edges of the wound toward the center. A special dressing is placed in the wound or over a graft or flap, which removes fluids from the wound and stimulates growth of healthy granulation tissue. The procedure is used for acute and traumatic wounds and pressure ulcers or chronic open wounds, such as diabetic ulcers, meshed grafts, and skin flaps. You may assist the physician or wound care specialist with the procedure.

CONTRAINDICATIONS
- Fistulas that involve organs or body cavities
- Necrotic tissue with eschar
- Untreated osteomyelitis
- Malignant wounds
- Use cautiously in patients with active bleeding, patients undergoing anticoagulant therapy, and in patients with a history of difficult wound hemostasis.

EQUIPMENT
Waterproof trash bag ● goggles ● gown, if indicated ● emesis basin ● normal saline solution ● clean gloves ● sterile gloves ● sterile scissors or a scalpel ● linen-saver pad ● 35-ml piston syringe with 19G catheter ● reticulated foam ● fenestrated tubing ● evacuation tubing ● skin protectant wipe ● transparent occlusive air-permeable drape ● evacuation canister ● vacuum unit

PREPARATION OF EQUIPMENT
- Assemble the VAC device at the bedside.
- Negative pressure is set according to the physician's order (25 to 200 mm Hg).

ESSENTIAL STEPS
- Check the physician's order for the dressing change and for any preprocedure analgesics to be administered.
- Verify the patent's identity using two patient identifiers, such as the patient's name and identification number.
- Reinforce the explanation of the procedure, provide privacy, and wash your hands.
- If necessary, put on a gown and goggles to protect yourself from wound drainage and contamination.
- Place a linen-saver pad under the patient to catch spills.
- Position the patient to allow maximum wound exposure, and place the emesis basin under the wound to collect drainage.
- Put on clean gloves; remove the soiled dressing and discard.

RED FLAG If the dressing being removed is a VAC dressing, ensure that the suction is off before removing the dressing to

*prevent damage to a healing wound bed and discomfort to the patient.
If the dressing is difficult to remove, normal saline solution is used to
loosen it from the wound bed.*

■ The physician or wound care specialist will:
  - attach the 19G catheter to the 35-ml piston syringe and irri-
    gate the wound thoroughly using normal saline solution
  - clean the area around the wound with normal saline solution;
    wipe intact skin with a skin protectant wipe and allow it to
    dry
  - remove and discard soiled gloves and put on sterile gloves
  - cut the foam to the shape and measurement of the wound us-
    ing sterile scissors or a scalpel (More than one piece may be
    needed to get the right size.)
  - carefully place the foam in the wound
  - place the fenestrated tubing into the center of the foam; this
    delivers negative pressure to the wound
  - place the transparent occlusive air-permeable drape over the
    foam, enclosing the foam and the tubing together
  - remove and discard soiled gloves
  - connect the free end of the fenestrated tubing to the tubing
    that's connected to the evacuation canister
  - turn on the vacuum unit and ensure that the dressing is occlu-
    sive by observing for the effects of the vacuum pressure on the
    dressing; the dressing should compress when the suction is
    turned on.

RED FLAG *If the dressing doesn't compress when suction is
applied, listen for an air leak in the dressing. Use occlusive
dressing strips to cover any holes in the occlusive dressing that may
be causing a leak. If you can't detect the exact location of the leak, the
area of the occlusive dressing that's over the sponge and the tubing
may need to be reinforced.*

■ When the procedure is finished, make sure the patient is comfortable.
■ Dispose of drainage, solution, linen-saver pad, and trash bag.
  Clean and dispose of soiled equipment and supplies according to
  guidelines.

SPECIAL CONSIDERATIONS

■ The dressing is changed every 48 hours; try to coordinate the
  dressing change with the physician's visit so he can inspect the
  wound.
■ Measure the amount of drainage every shift.

- Audible and visual alarms alert you if the unit is tipped greater than 45 degrees, the canister is full, the dressing has an air leak, or the canister becomes dislodged; make sure these alarms are working. Notify the wound care specialist and physician of problems.
- Reinforce the explanation of the procedure to the patient and answer questions.
- Depending on the location of the wound and the physician's orders, the patient may need to maintain bed rest during vacuum therapy. Provide support to the patient as needed.

COMPLICATIONS
Cleaning and care of wounds may temporarily increase the patient's pain and the risk of infection.

DOCUMENTATION
- Document the frequency and duration of therapy.
- Note who performed the procedure, the amount of negative pressure applied, the size and condition of the wound, and the patient's response to treatment.

Wound dehiscence and evisceration care

Surgical wounds usually heal well; however, the edges of a wound may fail to join or may separate after apparently healing normally. This may lead to more serious complications of evisceration, in which a portion of the viscera (usually a bowel loop) protrudes through the incision. Evisceration can lead to peritonitis and septic shock. Dehiscence and evisceration are most likely to occur 6 or 7 days after surgery, when sutures may have been removed and the patient can cough easily and breathe deeply—which strain the incision. (See *Recognizing dehiscence and evisceration,* page 266.)

These conditions may be caused by poor nutrition (from inadequate intake or conditions such as diabetes mellitus) or chronic pulmonary or cardiac disease and metastatic cancer (because the injured tissue doesn't get needed nutrients and oxygen). In addition, localized wound infection may limit closure, delay healing, and weaken the incision; and stress on the incision from coughing or vomiting may cause abdominal distention or severe stretching. (A midline abdominal incision poses a high risk of wound dehiscence.)

CONTRAINDICATIONS
None known.

Recognizing dehiscence and evisceration

In wound dehiscence, the layers of the surgical wound separate. With evisceration, the viscera (in this case, a bowel loop) protrude through the surgical incision.

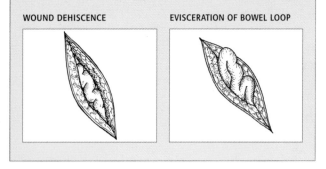

WOUND DEHISCENCE   EVISCERATION OF BOWEL LOOP

EQUIPMENT

Two sterile towels ● 1 L of sterile normal saline solution ● sterile irrigation set, including a basin, a solution container, and a 50-ml catheter-tip syringe ● several large abdominal dressings ● sterile, waterproof drape ● linen-saver pads ● sterile gloves

If the patient will return to the operating room

All previous equipment ● I.V. administration set, I.V. fluids, and 18G I.V. catheter ● equipment for nasogastric (NG) intubation ● sedative ● suction apparatus

ESSENTIAL STEPS

- Provide emotional support.
- Remind the patient that he must stay in bed. If possible, stay with him while someone else notifies the physician and collects the necessary equipment.
- Place a linen-saver pad under him to keep sheets dry when you moisten the exposed viscera.
- Using sterile technique, unfold a sterile towel to create a sterile field.
- Open the package containing the irrigation set, and place the basin, solution container, and 50-ml syringe on the sterile field.

■ Open the bottle of normal saline solution and pour about 400 ml into the solution container and about 200 ml into the sterile basin.

■ Open several large abdominal dressings and place them on the sterile field.

■ Put on the sterile gloves and place one or two of the large abdominal dressings into the basin to saturate them with normal saline solution.

■ Gently place the moistened dressings over the exposed viscera; place a sterile, waterproof drape over the dressings to prevent the sheets from getting wet.

■ Moisten the dressings every hour by drawing normal saline solution into a syringe and squirting solution on the dressings.

■ When you moisten the dressings, inspect the color of the viscera.

RED FLAG If the viscera appears dusky or black, notify the supervising RN and physician immediately. With its blood supply interrupted, a protruding organ may become ischemic and necrotic.

■ Keep the patient on absolute bed rest in low Fowler's position (no more than 20 degrees' elevation) with his knees flexed to prevent injury and reduce stress on an abdominal incision.

■ Monitor the patient's pulse, respirations, blood pressure, and temperature every 15 minutes to detect shock.

■ Depending on circumstances, repair of dehiscence or evisceration may not be done at the bedside. If necessary, prepare the patient to return to the operating room and ensure informed consent is obtained.

■ Have an I.V. inserted with an 18G I.V. catheter, initiate I.V. infusion, and maintain the infusion.

■ Insert an NG tube and connect it to continuous or intermittent low suction.

RED FLAG NG intubation may make the patient gag or vomit, causing further evisceration; the physician may choose to have the NG tube inserted in the operating room with the patient under anesthesia.

RED FLAG To decrease the risk of aspiration during surgery, don't allow the patient to have anything by mouth.

■ Give preoperative drugs to the patient, or contact the registered nurse to give them.

■ Continue to reassure the patient while you prepare him for surgery.

SPECIAL CONSIDERATIONS
■ If you're caring for a postoperative patient who's at risk for poor healing, make sure he gets an adequate supply of protein, vitamins, and calories. Monitor his dietary deficiencies; discuss problems with the supervising RN.
■ Reinforce that the patient should practice good hygiene and handwashing.
■ Change wound dressings as ordered or when soiled and always use sterile technique.
■ Monitor the incision with each dressing change; if you recognize signs of infection, contact the supervising RN and physician.
■ If local infection develops, clean the wound as necessary to eliminate a buildup of purulent drainage.
■ Make sure bandages aren't so tight that they limit blood supply to the wound.
■ Reinforce the explanation of the procedures and reassure the patient before surgery.
■ Reinforce with the patient how to splint his incision during coughing and deep breathing to prevent dehiscence and evisceration.
■ Reinforce the dietary requirements during the healing stage and review the components of an appropriate diet.

COMPLICATIONS
Complications include infection, peritonitis, septic shock, and necrosis of the protruding bowel loop.

DOCUMENTATION
■ Note when the dehiscence or evisceration occurred.
■ Record the patient's activity preceding the event.
■ Document his condition, response to the event, and the time the physician was notified.
■ Describe the appearance of the wound or eviscerated organ; the amount, color, consistency, and odor of drainage; and nursing and physician actions taken.
■ Record vital signs.
■ Review care plans frequently and amend them to reflect nursing actions needed to promote proper healing.

Wound irrigation

Wound irrigation cleans tissues and flushes cell debris and drainage from an open wound. Wound irrigation helps the wound heal properly from the inside tissue layers outward to the skin surface and prevents premature surface healing over an abscess pocket or infected tract. Strict sterile technique is required. After irrigation, open wounds are usually packed to absorb additional drainage.

CONTRAINDICATIONS
None known.

EQUIPMENT
Waterproof trash bag ● linen-saver pad ● emesis basin ● clean gloves ● sterile gloves ● goggles ● gown, if indicated ● prescribed irrigant such as sterile normal saline solution ● sterile water ● soft rubber or plastic catheter ● sterile container ● materials as needed for wound care ● sterile irrigation and dressing set ● commercial wound cleaner (if ordered) ● piston syringe and rubber catheter or 35-ml syringe with 19G needle or catheter ● skin protectant wipe

PREPARATION OF EQUIPMENT
■ Assemble the equipment in the patient's room.
■ Check the expiration date on each sterile package, and inspect for tears.
■ Check the sterilization date and the date that each bottle of irrigating solution was opened; don't use a solution that's been open longer than 24 hours.
■ Using sterile technique, dilute the prescribed irrigant to the correct proportions with sterile water or normal saline solution.
■ Let the solution stand until it reaches room temperature, or warm it to 90° to 95° F (32.2° to 35° C).

⚠ *RED FLAG Never warm irrigating solutions, especially in the microwave. Warming may cause uneven heating and scald the patient's wound.*

■ Position the waterproof trash bag to avoid reaching across the sterile field or the wound when disposing of soiled items. Turn down the top of the trash bag to provide a wide opening, preventing contamination by touching the bag's edge.

ESSENTIAL STEPS
■ Check the physician's order for the wound irrigation and any pre-procedure analgesics to be given.
■ Verify the patent's identity using two patient identifiers, such as the patient's name and identification number.
■ Identify allergies to topical solutions or drugs.
■ Reinforce the explanation of the procedure to the patient, provide privacy, and position him for the procedure.

■ Place the linen-saver pad under him to catch spills.
■ Place the emesis basin below the wound so irrigating solution flows from the wound into the basin.
■ Wash your hands and put on gloves.
■ Put on a gown to protect yourself from wound drainage and contamination.
■ Remove the soiled dressing noting the amount, color, consistency, and odor of any drainage and the wound's size, depth, and appearance.
■ Discard the dressing and gloves in the trash bag.
■ Establish a sterile field with the equipment and supplies you'll need for irrigation and wound care.
■ Pour the prescribed amount of irrigating solution into a sterile container so you won't contaminate your sterile gloves later by picking up unsterile containers.
■ Put on sterile gloves, gown, and goggles.
■ Fill the syringe with irrigating solution.
■ Instill a slow, steady stream of irrigating solution into the wound until the syringe empties. (See *Irrigating a deep wound.*)
■ Make sure the solution reaches all areas of the wound and flows from the clean to the dirty area of the wound to prevent contamination of clean tissue.
■ Refill the syringe, and repeat irrigation.
■ Continue to irrigate the wound until you've given the prescribed amount of solution or until the solution returns clear.
■ Note the amount of solution given.
■ Keep the patient positioned to allow further wound drainage into the basin.
■ Clean the area around the wound with normal saline solution; wipe intact skin with a skin protectant wipe and allow it to dry to help prevent skin breakdown and infection.
■ Pack the wound, if ordered, and apply a sterile dressing.
■ Remove and discard your gloves, gown, and goggles.
■ Wash your hands.
■ Properly dispose of drainage, solutions, and the trash bag, and clean or dispose of soiled equipment and supplies.

RED FLAG To prevent contamination of other equipment, don't return unopened sterile supplies to the sterile supply cabinet.

SPECIAL CONSIDERATIONS
■ Try to coordinate wound irrigation with the physician's visit so he can assess the wound.
■ Use only the irrigant specified by the physician; others may be erosive or otherwise harmful.

Irrigating a deep wound

When preparing to irrigate a wound, use the prescribed irrigant, such as sterile normal saline, and a piston syringe (without a needle) and a rubber catheter to ensure low-pressure irrigation. Irrigation may also be performed by attaching a 19G needle or catheter to a 35-ml syringe. This setup delivers an irrigation pressure of 8 psi, which is effective in cleaning the wound and reducing risk of trauma and wound infection. To prevent tissue damage, or intestinal perforation in an abdominal wound, avoid forcing the needle or catheter into the wound. Irrigate the wound with gentle pressure until the solution returns clean. Position the emesis basin under the wound to collect remaining drainage.

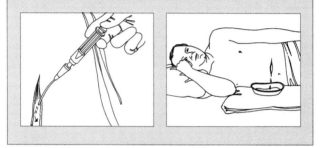

- Follow your facility's policy and Centers for Disease Control and Prevention guidelines concerning wound and skin precautions.
- Irrigate with a bulb syringe only if a piston syringe is unavailable. Use a bulb syringe cautiously because it doesn't deliver enough pressure to adequately clean the wound. If the wound is small or not particularly deep, you may use just the syringe for irrigation.
- If the wound must be irrigated at home, reinforce with the patient or a family member how to do it using strict sterile technique. Review the written instructions.
- Monitor the patient's or family member's demonstration of the proper technique.
- Help arrange for home health supplies and nursing visits, as appropriate.
- Reinforce that the patient should call his physician if he detects signs of infection.

COMPLICATIONS

Complications include wound infection, excoriation of the surrounding skin, pain, and wound trauma.

DOCUMENTATION
- Record the date and time of irrigation and amount and type of irrigant.
- Note the appearance of the wound and sloughing tissue or exudate.
- Document the amount of solution returned.
- Record skin care performed around the wound and dressings applied.
- Note the patient's tolerance of the treatment.

Wound management, surgical

Wound management procedures help prevent infection by stopping pathogens from entering the wound. The procedures promote patient comfort and protect the skin surface from maceration and excoriation caused by contact with irritating drainage. They also allow you to measure wound drainage to monitor healing and fluid and electrolyte balance. There are two primary methods of wound management: dressing and pouching. *Dressing* is preferred unless caustic or excessive drainage is compromising skin integrity. Lightly seeping wounds with drains and wounds with minimal purulent drainage can be managed with packing and gauze dressings. Some wounds, such as those that become chronic, may require an occlusive dressing. A wound with copious, excoriating drainage calls for *pouching* to protect the surrounding skin. If the patient has a surgical wound, monitor him and confer with the physician and registered nurse so the physician can order the appropriate dressing. Together, use the color of the wound to help determine which type of dressing should be applied. (See *Tailoring wound care to wound color.*)

Surgical wound management procedures require sterile technique and sterile supplies to prevent contamination. Change the dressing often enough to keep the skin dry.

CONTRAINDICATIONS
None known.

EQUIPMENT
Waterproof trash bag ● clean gloves ● sterile gloves ● gown and face shield or goggles, if indicated ● sterile 4″ × 4″ gauze pads ● large absorbent dressings, if indicated ● sterile cotton-tipped applicators ● sterile dressing set ● povidone-iodine swabs or other antiseptic solution ● topical drug, if ordered ● adhesive or other tape ● soap and water ● skin protectant ● nonadherent pads ● collodion

Tailoring wound care to wound color

If your patient has an open wound, you can monitor how well it's healing by inspecting its color, which you can then use to guide management of the wound.

RED WOUNDS

Red indicates normal healing. When a wound begins to heal, a layer of pale pink granulation tissue covers the wound bed. As it thickens, it becomes beefy red.

Cover a red wound, keep it moist and clean, and protect it from trauma. Use a transparent dressing (such as Tegaderm or Op-site), a hydrocolloidal dressing (such as DuoDERM), or a gauze dressing moistened with sterile normal saline solution or impregnated with petroleum jelly or an antibiotic.

YELLOW WOUNDS

Yellow is the color of exudate produced by microorganisms in an open wound. Exudate usually appears whitish yellow, creamy yellow, yellowish green, or beige. Water content influences shade: Dry exudate appears darker.

If the wound is yellow, clean it and remove exudate using high-pressure irrigation; then cover it with a moist dressing. Use absorptive

products (for example, Debrisan beads and paste) or a moist gauze dressing with or without an antibiotic. You may also use hydrotherapy with whirlpool or irrigation.

BLACK WOUNDS

Black, the least healthy color, signals necrosis and requires debridement. Dead, avascular tissue slows healing and provides a site for microorganisms to proliferate.

After removing dead tissue, apply a dressing to keep the wound moist and guard against external contamination. As ordered, use enzyme products, surgical debridement, hydrotherapy with whirlpool or irrigation, or a moist gauze dressing.

MULTICOLORED WOUNDS

You may note two or even all three colors in a wound. In this case, classify the wound according to the least healthy color present. For example, if the wound is red and yellow, classify it as a yellow wound.

spray or acetone-free adhesive remover ● sterile normal saline solution ● graduated container ● Montgomery straps, a fishnet tube elasticized dressing support, or a T-binder (optional)

For a wound with a drain

Sterile scissors ● sterile 4″ × 4″ gauze pads without cotton lining ● sump drain ● ostomy pouch or another collection bag ● sterile precut tracheostomy pads or drain dressings ● adhesive tape (paper or silk tape if patient is hypersensitive) ● surgical mask

For pouching a wound

Collection pouch with drainage port ● sterile gloves ● skin protectant ● sterile gauze pads

PREPARATION OF EQUIPMENT

■ Monitor the patient's condition and identify allergies to adhesive tape, povidone-iodine or other topical solutions, or drugs.
■ Assemble the equipment in his room.
■ Check the expiration date on each sterile package and inspect for tears.
■ Put the waterproof trash bag near the patient to avoid reaching across the sterile field or the wound when disposing of soiled items.
■ Turn down the top of the trash bag to provide a wide opening and prevent contamination of instruments or gloves by touching the bag's edge.

ESSENTIAL STEPS

■ Verify the patent's identity using two patient identifiers, such as the patient's name and identification number.
■ Reinforce the explanation of the procedure to the patient.
■ Check the physician's order for specific wound care and preprocedure analgesics to be administered.
■ Note the location of surgical drains to avoid dislodging them during the procedure.
■ Provide privacy, position the patient as necessary, and expose the wound site.
■ Wash your hands and put on a gown, clean gloves, and goggles or a face shield, if necessary.
■ Slowly remove the soiled dressing.

RED FLAG Hold the patient's skin and pull the tape or dressing toward the wound. This protects the newly formed tissue and prevents stress on the incision. Moisten the tape with acetone-free adhesive remover, if necessary, to make tape removal less painful (particularly if the skin is hairy). If the gauze adheres to the wound, moisten it with sterile normal saline solution to loosen it. Don't apply solvents to the incision; they can contaminate the wound.

■ Observe the dressing for amount, type, color, and odor of drainage.
■ Discard the dressing and gloves in the waterproof trash bag.

Caring for the wound

■ Wash your hands.

■ Establish a sterile field with the equipment and supplies you'll need for suture-line care and dressing change, including a sterile dressing set and povidone-iodine swabs.

■ If the physician has ordered ointment, squeeze the needed amount onto the sterile field.

■ If using an antiseptic from an unsterile bottle, pour the antiseptic cleaning agent into a sterile container so you won't contaminate your gloves.

■ Put on sterile gloves.

■ Saturate the sterile gauze pads with the prescribed cleaning agent.

RED FLAG Avoid using cotton balls. They may shed fibers in the wound, causing irritation, infection, or adhesion.

■ If ordered, obtain a wound culture; then proceed to clean the wound.

■ Pick up the moistened gauze pad or swab and squeeze out excess solution.

■ Working from the top of the incision, wipe once to the bottom, and then discard.

■ Wipe a second moistened pad from top to bottom in a vertical path next to the incision.

■ Continue to work outward from the incision in lines running parallel to it.

RED FLAG Always wipe from the clean area toward the less clean area (usually from top to bottom) and use each gauze pad or swab for only one stroke to prevent contamination. The suture line is cleaner than adjacent skin and the top of the suture line is usually cleaner than the bottom where drainage collects.

■ Use sterile cotton-tipped applicators for efficient cleaning of tight-fitting wire sutures, deep and narrow wounds, or wounds with pockets.

■ Wipe only once with each applicator.

■ If the patient has a surgical drain, clean the drain's surface last.

■ Moist drainage promotes bacterial growth; the drain is considered the most contaminated area. Clean the skin around the drain by wiping in half or full circles from the drain site outward.

■ Clean all areas of the wound to wash away debris, pus, blood, and necrotic material. Try not to disturb sutures or irritate the incision.

■ Clean to at least 1″ (2.5 cm) beyond the end of the new dressing. If you aren't applying a new dressing, clean to at least 2″ (5.1 cm) beyond the incision.

■ Monitor the edges of the incision to ensure that they're lined up properly, and monitor for signs of infection (heat, redness, swelling, induration, and odor), dehiscence, or evisceration.

🚩 *RED FLAG If you note signs of infection or the patient reports pain at the wound site, notify the supervising RN and physician.*

■ Irrigate the wound.
■ Wash the skin surrounding the wound with soap and water, and pat dry using a sterile 4″ × 4″ gauze pad.

🚩 *RED FLAG Avoid oil-based soap; it may interfere with pouch adherence. Apply prescribed topical drugs.*

■ Apply a skin protectant if needed.
■ If ordered, pack the wound with gauze pads or strips folded to fit, using sterile forceps.

🚩 *RED FLAG Avoid using cotton-lined gauze pads. Cotton fibers can adhere to the wound surface and cause complications.*

■ Gently pack the wound using the wet-to-damp method. Soaking the packing material in solution and wringing it out so it's slightly moist provides a moist wound environment that absorbs debris and drainage. Removing the packing won't disrupt new tissue.

🚩 *RED FLAG Don't pack the wound tightly. It may cause wound damage.*

Applying a fresh gauze dressing

■ Place sterile 4″ × 4″ gauze pads at the center of the wound, and move progressively outward to the edges of the wound site.
■ Extend the gauze at least 1″ (2.5 cm) beyond the incision in each direction, and cover the wound evenly with enough sterile dressings (usually two or three layers) to absorb drainage until the next dressing change.
■ Use large absorbent dressings to form outer layers, if needed, to provide greater absorbency.
■ Secure the edges of the dressing to the patient's skin with strips of tape to maintain sterility of the wound site, or secure the dressing with a T-binder or Montgomery straps to prevent skin excoriation, which may occur with repeated tape removal necessitated by frequent dressing changes.
■ If the wound is on a limb, secure the dressing with a fishnet tube elasticized dressing support.
■ Make sure the patient is comfortable.
■ Properly dispose of the solutions and trash bag. Clean or discard soiled equipment and supplies according to facility policy.

RED FLAG *Don't return unopened sterile supplies to the sterile supply cabinet; this could cross-contaminate other equipment.*

Dressing a wound with a drain

■ Prepare a drain dressing by using sterile scissors to cut a slit in a sterile 4″ × 4″ gauze pad.

■ Fold the pad in half; then cut inward from the center of the folded edge.

■ Don't use a cotton-lined gauze pad. Cutting the gauze opens the lining and releases cotton fibers into the wound.

■ Prepare a second pad the same way, or use commercially precut gauze.

■ Press one folded pad close to the skin around the drain so that the tubing fits into the slit. Press the second folded pad around the drain from the opposite direction so that the two pads encircle the tubing.

■ Layer as many uncut sterile 4″ × 4″ gauze pads or large absorbent dressings around the tubing as needed to absorb expected drainage. Tape the dressing in place, or use a T-binder or Montgomery straps.

Pouching a wound

■ If the patient's wound is draining heavily or if drainage may damage the surrounding skin, apply a pouch.

■ Measure the wound. Cut an opening ⅜″ (0.3 cm) larger than the wound in the facing of the collection pouch.

■ Apply a skin protectant as needed.

■ Plan to position the drainage port so that gravity facilitates drainage.

■ Make sure the drainage port at the bottom of the pouch is closed firmly to prevent leaks.

■ Gently press the contoured pouch opening around the wound, starting at its lower edge, to catch drainage.

■ To empty the pouch, put on gloves and a face shield or mask and goggles in case of splashing.

■ Insert the bottom of the pouch halfway into a graduated biohazard container, and open the drainage port. Note the color, consistency, odor, and amount of fluid.

■ If ordered, obtain a culture specimen and send it to the laboratory immediately.

■ Follow Centers for Disease Control and Prevention standard precautions when handling infectious drainage.

■ Wipe the bottom of the pouch and drainage port with a gauze pad and reseal the port.
■ Change the pouch only if it leaks or fails to adhere.

SPECIAL CONSIDERATIONS

■ If the patient has two wounds in the same area, cover each wound separately with layers of sterile 4″ × 4″ gauze pads. Cover each site with a large absorbent dressing secured to the patient's skin with tape.
■ Don't use a single large absorbent dressing to cover both sites because drainage quickly saturates a pad, promoting cross-contamination.
■ Don't pack the wound too tightly.
■ Avoid overlapping damp packing onto surrounding skin because it macerates the intact tissue.
■ To save time when dressing a wound with a drain, use precut tracheostomy pads or drain dressings to fit around the drain.
■ If the patient is sensitive to adhesive tape, use paper or silk tape.
■ Use a surgical mask to cradle a chin or jawline dressing.
■ If ordered, use a collodion spray or similar topical protectant instead of a gauze dressing.
■ If a sump drain isn't adequately collecting wound secretions, reinforce it with an ostomy pouch or another collection bag.
■ Use waterproof tape to strengthen a spot on the top and front of the pouch near the adhesive opening; then cut a small "X" in the tape. Feed the drain catheter into the pouch through the "X" cut.
■ Seal the cut around the tubing with more waterproof tape; then connect the tubing to the suction pump.
■ If you use more than one collection pouch for a wound or wounds, record drainage volume separately for each pouch.
■ Avoid using waterproof material over the dressing.
■ Many physicians prefer to change the first postoperative dressing themselves so they can assess the incision; don't change the primary dressing unless you have specific instructions.
■ If you have no such order and drainage comes through the dressings, reinforce the dressing with fresh sterile gauze. Request an order to change the dressing, or ask the physician to change it as soon as possible.
■ A reinforced dressing shouldn't remain in place longer than 24 hours because it's a medium for bacterial growth.
■ For the recent postoperative patient or a patient with complications, check the dressing every 15 to 30 minutes or as ordered.

For the patient with a properly healing wound, check the dressing at least once every 8 hours.

■ If the dressing becomes wet from the outside, replace it as soon as possible to prevent wound contamination.
■ Reinforce with the patient instructions about the wound care methods he'll use after discharge.
■ Remind him of the importance of using sterile technique.
■ Review instructions on how to monitor the wound for infection and other complications.
■ Reinforce with the patient how to change dressings.
■ Review the written instructions for procedures to be performed at home with the patient.

COMPLICATIONS

Complications include allergic reactions; skin redness, rash, or excoriation; infection; and skin tears.

DOCUMENTATION

■ Note special or detailed wound care instructions and pain management steps on the care plan.
■ Note the date, time, and type of wound management procedure.
■ Record a description of the soiled dressing and the amount of packing removed.
■ Document the wound appearance (including size, condition of margins, and presence of necrotic tissue) and odor (if present).
■ Note the type, color, consistency, and amount of drainage (for each wound) and the presence and location of drains.
■ Note additional procedures performed, such as irrigation, packing, or application of a topical drug.
■ Document the type of dressing or pouch applied and the amount of packing used.
■ Record the patient's tolerance of the procedure.

Cultural considerations in patient care

Regardless of the setting in which you work, as a health care professional you'll typically interact with a diverse, multicultural patient population and you should base your care plan on the overall needs of the patient and his family. Generally, each culture has its own unique set of beliefs about health and illness, dietary practices, and other matters that you should consider when providing care.

Although negative stereotyping of different cultures must be avoided, it's important to learn about representative characteristics of different groups. However, you should be aware that people have widely varying beliefs that are sometimes based only in part on cul-

CULTURAL GROUP	HEALTH CARE BELIEF AND ILLNESS PHILOSOPHY
African Americans	• May believe that illness is related to supernatural causes • May seek advice and remedies from faith or folk healers • May show stoic response to pain until it's unbearable and then seek emergency care • May be family oriented; customary for many family members to remain with a dying patient in the hospital • May express grief by crying, screaming, praying, singing, and reading scripture
Arab Americans (major populations include those from Egypt, Iran, Iraq, Lebanon, Palestine, and Syria)	• May remain silent about some health problems such as sexually transmitted diseases, substance abuse, mental illness • A devout Muslim may interpret illness as the will of Allah, a test of faith, representing a type of fatalistic view • May rely on ritual cures or alternative therapies before seeing a health care provider • May have strong respect for the elderly and feel obliged to take care of elderly relatives • May express pain freely

tural heritage. Health care professionals should try to understand each person and be sensitive to and respectful of individual beliefs.

This appendix summarizes some health care beliefs and practices relating to dietary, communication, family roles, death rituals, health care practices, and folk health practices for five cultural groups that are common in the United States. These include African Americans, Arab Americans, Asian Americans, Latino Americans, and Native Americans. The predominant Western culture health care beliefs and practices are also summarized.

DIETARY PRACTICES	OTHER CONSIDERATIONS
● May have food restrictions based on religious beliefs (such as not eating pork, if Muslim) ● Have a higher incidence of high blood pressure and obesity, which may be diet related ● High incidence of lactose intolerance with difficulty digesting milk and milk products ● May view cooked greens as good for health ● Traditional "soul" food diet is high in protein and fat	● Predominant values: Family bonding, matriarchal, present orientation, and spiritual orientation ● Tend to be affectionate, as shown by touching and hugging friends and loved ones ● Many Muslim women must keep their heads covered at all times ● Primary religions: Baptist and other Protestant denominations, Muslim (Islam)
● May choose foods based on the humoral theory of balancing hot and cold ● May prefer dairy products, rice, and wheat breads ● May avoid pork and alcohol if Muslim	● Predominant values: Family patriarchal and hierarchical, respect for elders, modesty, respectability, and politeness ● Muslim women may avoid eye contact as a show of modesty ● Many Muslim women wear the traditional hijab (head cover) ● Respect for higher education and advanced degrees

CULTURAL GROUP	HEALTH CARE BELIEF AND ILLNESS PHILOSOPHY
Arab Americans *(continued)*	● After death, the family or community members may want to prepare the body by washing and wrapping the body in unsewn white cloth ● Postmortem examinations are discouraged unless required by law
Asian Americans **(major populations include those from Cambodia, China, India, Indonesia, Korea, Pakistan, Phillipines, Thailand, and Vietnam)**	● Asian Americans have differing health views depending in part on their particular subculture – Chinese: May believe illness results when a person fails to act in harmony with nature, such as yin and yang – Filipino: May believe dying is God's plan and that neither the client nor the health care provider should interfere with God's will – Korean: May adhere to traditional values that dictate that client should die at home – Japanese: May believe that illness is karma, resulting from behavior in the current life or a past life ● May value ability to endure pain and grief with silent stoicism ● Typically family oriented; extended family should be involved in care of dying patient
Latino Americans **(major populations include those from the Caribbean, Central and South America, and Mexico)**	● May view illness as a sign of weakness, punishment for evil doing or retribution for shameful behavior ● May use the terms "hot" and "cold" in reference to vital elements needed to restore equilibrium to the body ● May consult with a curandero (healer) or voodoo priest (Caribbean) ● May view pain as a necessary part of life and believe that enduring pain is a sign of strength (especially men) ● May have open expression of grief, such as praying for the dead, saying the rosary ● May use various amulets to protect individual from evil ● Family members are typically involved in all aspects of decision making such as terminal illness

DIETARY PRACTICES	**OTHER CONSIDERATIONS**
● Islamic patients observe month-long fast of Ramadan (begins approximately mid October); those who are suffering chronic illness and women who are pregnant, breast-feeding, or menstruating don't fast ● May avoid mixing milk and fish, sweet and sour, or hot and cold ● May avoid using ice in drinks ● May believe that hot soup can help recovery	● Use same-sex family members as interpreters ● Preventive care among adults isn't highly valued ● Primary religions: Catholic, Greek Orthodox, Muslim (Islam), Protestant
● Hot/cold theory (yin and yang) often involved. Example: Curing a "hot" disease such as arthritis may require cold foods or medicines ● Hindu religious food practices include refraining from eating meat from cows; some are lacto-vegetarians eating only milk products and vegetables ● Chinese patients may use an herbalist or acupuncturist before seeking medical help; may eat rice with most meals and may use chopsticks ● Sodium intake is generally high because of salted and dried foods and use of condiments	● Predominant values: Group orientation, submission to authority, respect for elders, respect for past, modesty, conformity, and tradition ● May believe that prolonged eye contact is rude and an invasion of privacy ● Tend to be very modest; prefer same sex clinicians ● May nod without necessarily understanding (especially elderly Japanese patients) ● May prefer to maintain a comfortable physical distance between the patient and the health care provider ● Primary Religions: Buddhist, Catholic, Confucianism, Hindu and Islam (India), Protestant, Shinto (Japanese), Taoism, Zen Buddhism
● May use herbal teas and soup to aid in recuperation ● Traditional diet is basically vegetarian with emphasis on corn, corn products, beans, rice, and breads ● Select beans and tortillas are staples and may be eaten at every meal ● Typically eat a lot of fresh fruits and vegetables; however, variety in diet may be limited ● High prevalence of obesity, particularly central obesity, that raises the risk of diabetes and heart disease	● Predominant values: Group emphasis, extended family, fatalism, present orientation ● May have fatalistic view of life ● May see no reason to submit to mammograms or vaccinations ● May need private room where grief can be expressed openly ● May be modest (especially women) ● Use same sex family members as interpreters ● Primary religion: Roman Catholic

CULTURAL GROUP	HEALTH CARE BELIEF AND ILLNESS PHILOSOPHY
Native Americans	● May turn to a medicine man to determine the true cause of an illness, such as why a person is out of harmony with nature ● May value the ability to endure pain or grief with silent stoicism ● May view death as part of life cycle ● Burial practices vary among tribal groups. Example: Navajos fear death and distance themselves from death and may avoid touching a dead or dying person. ● May believe that the spirit of a dying person can't leave his body until the family is there ● Grief tends to be family oriented with all members assuming roles in the grieving process
Western culture (primarily of European background)	● May value technology almost exclusively in the struggle to conquer disease ● May have strong shared belief in the biomedical approach, which may result in serious barriers to communication with other cultures who choose to use alternative or complementary therapies ● Health is generally understood to be the absence, minimization, or control of disease processes ● Hospitalization may foster an atmosphere that requires the patient and family to be compliant, dependent, and vulnerable to get needs met ● Health care emphasis is shifting from treating diseases to disease prevention and health promotion

DIETARY PRACTICES

- Diet may be deficient in vitamin D and calcium because many suffer from lactose intolerance or don't drink milk
- Obesity and diabetes are major health concerns
- Herbs are used in the treatment of many illnesses to cleanse the body of ill spirits or poisons

OTHER CONSIDERATIONS

- Predominant values: Bonding to family or group, sharing with others, present orientation, extended family, cooperation and acceptance of nature
- May divert their eyes to the floor when they are praying or paying attention
- Raised to be reserved and noncommittal, may respond to assessment questions with silence or monosyllables
- Belief system: Characterized by intense relationship with nature

---

- Heath care facilities frequently have standard dietary guidelines, which may consider cultural variations
- Eating utensils primarily consist of knife, fork, and spoon
- Three daily meals is typical
- Values convenience and may substitute ready-to-eat (fast food) items, which are generally low in nutrition and health benefits; meals eaten out tend to be higher in calories, fat, and sodium
- Growing incidence of obesity

- Predominant values: Independence, self-reliance and individualism, resistance to authority, nuclear or blended family, innovation, emphasis on youth, future orientation, competition
- Belief systems widely varied

Cardiopulmonary resuscitation

Adults or adolescents

Action	Implementation
Check for unresponsiveness	Gently shake and shout, "Are you OK?"
Call for help and call 9-1-1	Immediately call for help and activate the emergency response numbers (9-1-1). If a second rescuer is available, send him to get help and an automated external defibrillator (AED) if available. Start cardiopulmonary resuscitation (CPR), if indicated. If likely asphyxial arrest, perform 5 cycles (about 2 minutes) of CPR before activating EMS.
Position patient	Place patient in a supine position on a hard, flat surface.
Open airway	Use head-tilt, chin-lift maneuver unless contraindicated by trauma.
If you suspect trauma	Open airway using the jaw-thrust method.
Check for adequate breathing	Look, listen, and feel for 10 seconds.

Action	Implementation
Perform ventilations	Give two breaths initially, then one every 5 to 6 seconds at 1 second/breath.
If chest doesn't rise	Reposition and reattempt ventilations.
Check pulse	Palpate the carotid pulse for no more than 10 seconds.
Start compressions Placement	If no pulse, place both hands, one atop the other, on the lower half of the sternum, between the nipples with elbows locked, and use a straight up-and-down motion without losing contact with the chest.
Depth	One-third the depth of the chest or 1½″ to 2″ (3.5 to 5 cm).
Rate	100/minute.
Compression:ventilation ratio	30:2 (if intubated: Continuous chest compressions at 100/minute without pauses for ventilation. Ventilations at 8 to 10 breaths/minute).
Check pulse	Palpate for carotid pulse after 2 minutes of CPR and as appropriate thereafter. Minimize interruptions in chest compressions.
Use AED	Apply as soon as available, and follow prompts. Provide 2 minutes of CPR after the first shock is delivered, before activating the AED to analyze the rhythm again and attempt another shock.

Choking

SIGNS AND SYMPTOMS
- Grabbing throat with hand
- Inability to speak
- Weak, ineffective coughing
- High-pitched sounds while inhaling

INTERVENTIONS

1. Ask the person, "Are you choking? Can you speak?" Assess for airway obstruction. Don't intervene if the person is coughing forcefully and can speak; a strong cough can dislodge the object.

2. Stand behind the person and wrap your arms around his waist. (If the person is pregnant or obese, wrap your hands around the chest.)

3. Make a fist with one hand, and place the thumb side of your fist just above the person's navel and well below the sternum.

4. Grasp your fist with your other hand.

5. Perform quick, upward and inward thrusts with your fist. (Perform chest thrusts for pregnant or obese persons.)

6. Continue thrusts until the object is dislodged or the victim loses consciousness.

If the victim loses consciousness, activate the emergency response number and begin cardiopulmonary resuscitation. Each time you open the airway to deliver rescue breaths, look in the mouth and remove any object you see. Never perform a blind finger sweep.

Web resources

Advance News Magazine for LPNs
www.advanceforlpns.com

Agency for Healthcare Research and Quality
www.ahrq.gov

Allnurses.com
www.allnurses.com

American Burn Association
www.ameriburn.org

American Cancer Society
www.cancer.org

American Diabetes Association
www.diabetes.org

American Heart Association
www.americanheart.org

American Holistic Nurses Association
www.ahna.org

American Lung Association
www.lungusa.org

American Pain Society
www.ampainsoc.org

Centers for Disease Control and Prevention
www.cdc.gov

Infusion Nurses Society
www.ins1.org

LPN Central – The Practical Nurse's Station
www.lpncentral.com

National Association for Practical Nurse Education
  & Service, Inc.
www.napnes.org

National Institutes of Health
www.nih.gov

National Kidney Foundation
www.kidney.org

National League for Nursing
www.nln.org

National Library of Medicine
www.ncbi.nlm.nih.gov/PubMed

Wound Ostomy & Continence Nurses Society
www.wocn.org

Selected references

American Association of Critical Care Nurses. *AACN Procedure Manual for Critical Care,* 5th ed. Edited by Lynn-McHale Wiegand, D.J., and Carlson, K.K. Philadelphia: W.B. Saunders Co., 2005.

Baldwin, K.M. "How to Prevent and Treat Pressure Ulcers," *LPN2005* 1(2):18-25, March-April 2005.

Comprehensive Accreditation Manual for Hospitals. Oakbrook Terrace, Ill.: Joint Commission on Accreditation of Healthcare Organizations, 2005.

ECG Interpretation: An Incredibly Easy Pocket Guide. Philadelphia: Lippincott Williams & Wilkins, 2006.

Evans-Smith, P. *Taylor's Clinical Nursing Skills: A Nursing Process Approach.* Philadelphia: Lippincott Williams & Wilkins, 2005.

Fast Facts for Nurses. Philadelphia: Lippincott Williams & Wilkins, 2004.

Fauci, A.S., et al. *Harrison's Principles of Internal Medicine,* 16th ed. New York: McGraw-Hill Book Co., 2005.

Guidelines for Isolation Precautions in Hospitals. Atlanta: Centers for Disease Control and Prevention, November 2002.

Hess, C.T. *Clinical Guide Wound Care,* 5th ed. Philadelphia: Lippincott Williams & Wilkins, 2005.

Ignatavicius, D.D., and Workmann, M.L. *Medical-Surgical Nursing Critical Thinking for Collaborative Care,* 5th ed. Philadelphia: W.B. Saunders Co., 2005.

Kaufman, M.W., and Pahl, D.W. "Vacuum-assisted Closure Therapy: Wound Care and Nursing Implications," *Dermatology Nursing* 15(4):317-25, August 2003.

National Patient Safety Goals. Oakbrook Terrace, Ill: Joint Commission on Accreditation of Healthcare Organizations, 2006.

Neal, L.J., and Guillett, S.E. *Care of the Adult with a Chronic Illness or Disability: A Team Approach.* St. Louis: Elsevier Mosby, 2004.

Nurse's Quick Check: Skills. Philadelphia: Lippincott Williams & Wilkins, 2006.

Poe, S.S., et al. "An Evidence-based Approach to Fall Risk Assessment, Prevention and Management: Lessons Learned," *Journal of Nursing Care Quality* 20(2):107-16, April-June 2005.

Rakel, R.E., and Bope, E.T., eds. *Conn's Current Therapy 2005.* Philadelphia: W.B. Saunders Co., 2005.

Smeltzer, S.C., and Bare, B.G. *Brunner and Suddarth's Textbook of Medical-Surgical Nursing,* 10th ed. Philadelphia: Lippincott Williams & Wilkins, 2004.

Thibodeau, G.A., and Patton, K.T. *The Human Body in Health and Disease,* 4th ed. St. Louis: Elsevier Mosby, 2005.

Timby, B.K. *Fundamental Nursing Skills and Concepts,* 8th ed. Philadelphia: Lippincott Williams & Wilkins, 2005.

Timby, B.K., and Smith, N.E. *Essentials of Nursing: Care of Adults and Children.* Philadelphia: Lippincott Williams & Wilkins, 2005.

Index

A

Abdomen
  auscultation of, 24-25
  inspection of, 24
  light palpation of, 25
Abdominal paracentesis assistance, 174-178. *See also* Paracentesis, abdominal.
  documenting, 178
  essential steps in, 175-177
  preparing equipment for, 175
  special considerations for, 177
Abuse, asking about, in health history, 7
Active listening as communication strategy, 3
Activities of daily living, health history and, 7-8
Add-a-line administration set. *See* Secondary I.V. line.
Administration sets, types of, 52i
Advance directive, 5
AED. *See* Automated external defibrillator.
African Americans, cultural considerations in patient care for, 282-283t
Airborne precautions, 31-34
  diseases that require, 32t
  essential steps in, 31-33
  special considerations for, 33-34

Air leak, assisting with locating, in thoracic drainage, 133-134
Airway obstruction
  as endotracheal tube complication, 108
  as mucus clearance complication, 119
  as tracheostomy care complication, 147
Airway patency, maintaining, during endotracheal tube care, 104
Alginate dressing, applying, to pressure ulcer, 254-255
Arab Americans, cultural considerations in patient care for, 282-285t
Arm amputation, aftercare for, 169. *See also* Stump and prosthesis care.
Arteriovenous fistula, hemodialysis access and, 218i
Arteriovenous graft, hemodialysis access and, 219i
Arteriovenous shunt, hemodialysis access and, 219i
Arteriovenous shunt care, 217-221
  contraindications for, 217
  documenting, 221
  equipment for, 219
  essential steps in, 219-221
  special considerations for, 221

---

i refers to an illustration; t refers to a table.

---

i refers to an illustration; t refers to a table.

i refers to an illustration; t refers to a table.

i refers to an illustration; t refers to a table.

i refers to an illustration; t refers to a table.

i refers to an illustration; t refers to a table.

---

i refers to an illustration; t refers to a table.

---

i refers to an illustration; t refers to a table.

Notes